The Politics of Physical Activity

Defining 'politics' as contests over ideas, values and visions about what a physically active society could be, this book uses critical analysis to challenge accepted truths about physical activity and therefore opens up a pathway to more effective, and more socially just, physical activity policy.

Critiquing global and national physical activity policies which are arguing for significant change to societies around the world, *The Politics of Physical Activity* presents empirical case studies to illustrate the political dimensions of advocating for physical activity promotion, including discussions of resourcing difficulties, conflicts of interest and opportunity costs. It explores physical activity as a multisectoral tool that is being applied to political ideas and policy goals as varied as education, sustainability and social cohesion, and asks what good physical activity really looks like.

This is important and provocative reading for any student, researcher, practitioner or policy maker with an interest in physical activity, public health or public policy.

Joe Piggin is Senior Lecturer in Sport Policy and Management in the School of Sport, Exercise and Health Sciences at Loughborough University, UK. Joe's research covers two main areas, namely sport policy translation into marketing and programmes, and physical activity policy. He is the co-editor (with Louise Mansfield and Mike Weed) of the *Routledge Handbook of Physical Activity Policy and Practice*.

Routledge Research in Physical Activity and Health

The *Routledge Research in Physical Activity and Health* series offers a multi-disciplinary forum for cutting-edge research in the broad area of physical activity, exercise and health. Showcasing the work of emerging and established scholars working in areas ranging from physiology and chronic disease, psychology and mental health to physical activity and health promotion and socio-economic and cultural aspects of physical activity participation, the series is an important channel for groundbreaking research in physical activity and health.

Physical Activity and the Gastro-Intestinal Tract
Responses in Health and Disease
Roy J. Shephard

Technology in Physical Activity and Health Promotion
Edited by Zan Gao

Physical Activity and the Abdominal Viscera
Responses in Health and Disease
Roy J. Shephard

Obesity: A Kinesiologist's Perspective
Roy J. Shephard

The Politics of Physical Activity
Joe Piggin

For more information about this series, please visit: www.routledge.com/sport/series/RRPAH

The Politics of Physical Activity

Joe Piggin

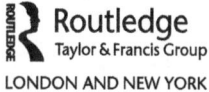

Routledge
Taylor & Francis Group

LONDON AND NEW YORK

First published 2019
by Routledge
2 Park Square, Milton Park, Abingdon, Oxon OX14 4RN

and by Routledge
52 Vanderbilt Avenue, New York, NY 10017

Routledge is an imprint of the Taylor & Francis Group, an informa business

British Library Cataloguing-in-Publication Data
A catalogue record for this book is available from the British Library

Library of Congress Cataloging-in-Publication Data
A catalog record has been requested for this book

ISBN: 978-0-367-25893-1 (hbk)
ISBN: 978-0-429-29038-1 (ebk)

Typeset in Times New Roman
by Wearset Ltd, Boldon, Tyne and Wear

Contents

1   Introduction

Physical activity is inherently political. Mixing empirical data, policy logic and ethical considerations, this book explores how physical activity is inherently political. The book includes:

*   A theoretical conceptualisation of physical activity as a multi-dimensional, multisectoral tool which is being applied to political ideas and policy goals.
*   Empirical case studies to illustrate the political dimensions of advocating for physical activity promotion, including discussions of resourcing difficulties, conflicts of interest and opportunity costs.
*   Critique of global and national physical activity policies which are arguing for significant change to societies around the world.

Governments, corporations, schools and local councils around the world are increasingly considering physical activity more seriously for various reasons. Physical activity is multidimensional and multisectoral. The ideas which inform physical activity promotion, from health, education and sustainability, to commerce, transport and morality are always in a state of flux – sometimes prioritised, at other times marginalised. Which ideas gain prominence and are emphasised in eventual decisions? Which and whose ideas are marginalised and omitted from policy discussions? These questions are important, since policy decisions (and non-decisions) about physical activity contribute to the dignity, values and life chances of individuals and communities. By understanding more about the political dimensions of physical activity, there will be space to develop less exploitative outcomes for the people affected by policy makers' decisions. There are opportunities to liberate populations to enjoy more active lives. However, to create such places and spaces, an understanding of the political dynamics that create physical structures and value systems about physical activity is required. This book examines a range of political elements which contribute to political thinking about physical activity and illuminates the forces which are using physical activity to achieve specific ends.

This book merges critical analysis with case studies to examine the *politics* inherent within the organisation, promotion and practice of physical activity. I take politics to involve contests over ideas, values and visions about what a physically active society could be.

Three factors make the politics of physical activity worthy of examination. First, the World Health Organisation's launch of its global physical activity strategy in 2018 has continued to elevate physical activity as an important health issue. Second, data from around the world continue to highlight the detrimental effects of poor health, often stemming from deepset inequalities. Physical activity is increasingly linked to issues of equity. Third, physical activity is a multidimensional, multisectoral practice, which is not comparable to a single health behaviour or disease. New insights into the politics which define, shape and influence physical activity is useful to the extent that it questions assumptions and strives to minimise unfair domination.

The text is structured as follows. Chapter 2, 'Contested definitions, histories and futures of physical activity', asks a range of questions about physical activity at a policy level. What values should be ascribed to physical activity? How much budget should be devoted to it? Who should benefit? At an individual level there are concerns about social justice, individual expression, liberty and surveillance. What physical activities are possible and permitted in a setting? What physical activities do people have a right to? How should people be judged with respect to the activities they partake in? This chapter situates the current concern about physical activity in its historical context and offers a variety of perspectives for critically analysing physical activity politics.

Chapter 3, 'Towards a physical activity discourse' argues that physical activity has developed into a specific *political discourse*. A model of the physical activity discourse is presented. This model examines how a variety of sub-discourses contribute to the political discourse through connections between essential, governing and sustaining discourses. A range of interest frames both feed into and are fed by the sustaining discourses of physical activity.

Chapter 4, 'Physical activity and the politics of knowledge' offers a critical analysis of a *Lancet* series on physical activity, which included the framing of physical inactivity as a 'pandemic'. Given the purported scale and significance of physical inactivity around the world, this chapter examines how the pandemic is rhetorically constructed and how various solutions are proposed. A governmentality lens is used to examine the continuity, coherence and appropriateness of ideas about physical activity.

The analysis demonstrates that within *The Lancet*, there is disunity about what is known about physical activity, problematic claims of 'abnormality' and contradictions in the proposed deployment of a systems approach to solve the problem.

Chapter 5, 'Physical activity and the politics of societal change', critically examines how we (people and communities) are encouraged to be physically active. How should our cities be organised? Which activities should be prescribed and encouraged? This chapter explores how archetypal thinking can influence physical activity policies. Through the analysis I argue that processes of homogenisation should not be understated. Physical activity promoters must tread carefully when elevating certain structures as ideal and certain activities as preferred or desired. Caution is warranted not only to avoid accusations of practices being imposed on a community and potential for marginalising traditional customs and practices within a local context, but also because some policy changes might be simply unachievable, and therefore inappropriate. To illustrate these points, there is an examination of how an apparently successful country's template (Finland) was attempted to be transposed onto another inactive country (the United Kingdom). Following this, a recent case study of the World Health Organisation's physical activity strategy is used to explore some of the values that inform international advocacy for physical activity promotion.

Chapter 6, 'Physical activity and the politics of junk food' moves the debate from state interventions to corporate involvement in physical activity promotion. Due to perceptions of a growing obesity issue, budgetary pressures and limited intervention effects, corporations have increasingly been framed as 'partners' in public health, working alongside government, councils and sports governing bodies. This chapter critically considers some of the ideas which dominate both the promotion of commercial partnerships in sport and physical activity promotion and resistance to them.

Chapter 7, 'Physical activity and the politics of corporate health promotion', continues the theme of corporate involvement, though this time with a case study of the Nike company, and its attempt to become involved in physical activity promotion (beyond selling shoes and clothes). This chapter examines three aspects of Nike's involvement in the global and UK conversation about physical activity. First, it examines Nike's involvement in building a theory about physical activity. Second, it considers Nike's alliance with a variety of state, civil society and professional organisations in the process of constructing the 'Designed To Move' lobby document. Third, the chapter examines Nike's attempted construction of a global physical activity 'movement' through the UK Physical Activity

Commission. By interrogating the political activities of the Nike corporation, we can see how physical activity is deployed to meet specific economic ends.

Chapter 8, 'Physical activity and the politics of risk' invokes a case study of recent and ongoing debate over the safety of collision sports such as rugby union. Rugby union is a popular sport in UK schools, and like countries such as Australia, New Zealand and South Africa, is often claimed to be the national sport. However, it has recently come under scrutiny for being too dangerous for children to play. England Rugby, the national governing body has been reluctant to remove the tackle element from the sport in schools. Instead, England Rugby emphasise the positive aspects that come from the sport. This chapter uses interactions between the author advocating for policy change and organisational responses to examine the political machinations of corporate entities promoting activities which are 'riskier' than others to children who may not be informed of the risks they are being exposed to.

Chapter 9, 'Conclusion: people, power and possibilities', concludes by considering the analysis within the text and looking to future political contests over physical activity. The various case studies presented here offer insight into one level of the politics of physical activity, yet it is clear there is a multitude of swirling conflicts about people's opportunities to be active, their understandings of what physical activity can and should include, and contests over resource allocation, from funding for everything from local bike lockers to cycle superhighways, students' options in physical education classes and expectations about what types of physical activities are socially acceptable, culturally appropriate, or even desired. This short chapter offers thoughts on what future political contests might arise about physical activity promotion, and how citizens and groups might organise to reject exploitative outcomes.

2 Contested definitions, histories and futures of physical activity

Concerns about physical activity are affecting many aspects of human life. Whether in homes, at schools, workplaces, in local communities, and in cities and countries, physical activity is becoming more intensely focused upon as a policy issue. In recent years there has been an escalating sense of urgency around improving population health through physical activity interventions. Various physical health outcomes such as the prevention of premature death are used to justify many interventions. However, physical activity and its adversary physical *inactivity* are complex phenomena. A range of other policy outcomes related to education, the economy, social cohesion and cultural development are also being linked with population-wide physical activity.

Physical activity has become a legitimate policy issue for which there are serious implications. At a *population level*, policy battles over scarce resources inevitably evoke concerns about equity, efficiency, sustainability, welfare and productivity. What values should be ascribed to physical activity? How much budget should be devoted to it? Who should benefit? At an *individual level* there are concerns about social justice, identity expression, liberty and surveillance. What physical activities are possible and permitted in a setting? What physical activities do people have a right to?

Physical activity is inherently political. Despite its growing association with 'health', physical activity is laden with a multitude of other values, including hierarchy, status and power, and contests and framing about inclusion and exclusion. So the promotion and provision of physical activity opportunities, and the ways that physical activity is embodied and manifested by participants, means it is never free from politics. These politics exist at various levels, from macro-politics – the dominant cultural values and priorities of a place, meso-level politics, its formal decision-making structures and processes, to micro-politics, involving those interpersonal relationships between people and their expectations, desires and values.

Simultaneously there is both synergy and conflict *within* and *between* these layers. For example, take a seemingly apolitical solitary walk around an urban neighbourhood. It would be influenced by feelings of safety or danger, the perceived threat of air pollution, and the social un/acceptability of someone walking alone. Rural spaces are just as political. A hike in the mountains is affected by a walker's existing resources to reach such a destination, and a region's government permitting such behaviour on rural land.

Most of the time the politics of physical activity is normalised. Physical environments tend not to become more inviting quickly or easily. A mixture of political values, limited resources, and the slow movement of the policy process means that hopes of everyone achieving physical activity guidelines are likely to be unachievably utopian. However, that should not stop us from trying to educate, facilitate and promote physical activity to populations. The plethora of quantified benefits associated with physical activity make for persuasive reading, and the humanistic values of freedom of movement (beyond immediate spaces as well as beyond borders) are important if humans are to flourish, find joy, and be free from unfair domination in their lives. Understanding more about the politics of physical activity, particularly in the ways it influences policy decisions, is an important consideration. It is the aim of this book to shed light onto often taken-for-granted and unquestioned political and policy dimensions of physical activity.

It is certainly the case that there is "strong evidence demonstrating the direct and indirect pathways by which physical activity prevents many of the major noncommunicable diseases (NCD) responsible for premature death and disability" (Bull and Bauman, 2011, p. 13). It is certainly true that "political changes, changes in government direction, and changing opportunities to profile active lifestyles" (Milton and Bauman, 2015, p. 1) are challenging for the up-scaling of physical activity policies and programmes. And it is true that "there has been an overall failure to scale up effective interventions at the population level" (Das and Horton, 2016, p. 1). While promoting physical activity can definitely be good to do (see Biddle and Mutrie, 2001), there are machinations beyond the success or failure of lobbying and programme development which are worth investigating. Critiques of *why* and *how* interventions are promoted can illuminate the interests that inform them. As will be seen in some of the case studies in this book, these interests are not always altruistic. Questions are also worth asking about archetypes of physical activity. Is there a best way to be physically active? What activities should people be encouraged to do? These answers might conflict with individuals' ideas about their bodies and their desired ways of being active.

What is physical activity? And what else could it be?

The starting point for this book is a challenge to a popular, official definition of physical activity. According to the World Health Organisation (WHO, 2017, 2018) physical activity is defined as "any bodily movement produced by skeletal muscles that requires energy expenditure". Commonly closely connected with this is the idea that "insufficient physical activity is a key risk factor for NCDs such as cardiovascular diseases, cancer and diabetes" (WHO, 2017). Thus, physical activity has come to be formally understood as being a finite set of body movements resulting in measurable energy expenditure and conferring physical health benefits. Of course, this definition is useful for the health and biomedical communities who seek to improve specific health outcomes, but is too narrow to capture what physical activity *is* for the people who partake in it, the advocates that promote it, and the organisations that arrange it. As well as potential health outcomes, there are various economic, cultural and environmental issues surrounding physical activity, meaning it is also a deeply political domain. I argue that the existing WHO definition is reductionist and exclusionary. It gives undue priority to the *anatomical/physiological*, at the exclusion of the *emotional, intellectual and political*. Therefore, other definitions of physical activity are possible, and inform the writing of this book.

An alternative definition might emphasise the individual lived experience as a core component of physical activity, drawing on ideas of struggle, joy, pain, pleasure, achievement. At a personal level, this is what we experience. Another definition could focus on the social, relational nature of physical activity. That is, physical activity is something we often do with other people, with outcomes and purposes not possible through solitary endeavour. And so at a personal and relational level, physical activity might be:

Political, Spiritual, Hysterical, Historic,
Exhaustive, Excruciating, Uninteresting, Protesting,
Sensual, Sexual, Risqué, Risky,
Arresting, Disarming, Investing, Resisting,
Painful, Painless, Subtle, Grand,
Curtailing, Surveilling, Obsessive, Compulsive,
Dialogical, Diabolical, Expensive, Discursive,
Ambient, Ambulant, Connecting, Correcting,
Wondrous, Wonderful, Unbearable, Uncomfortable,
Cathartic, Chaotic, Instructive, Destructive,
Balletic, Bathetic, Compulsory, Derisory,

Beneficial, Sacrificial, Moving, Reinforcing,
Instinctive, Artistic, Repulsive,
and/or
Oppressive.

Physical activity should not be thought of as one thing, or connected mainly with just one thing. For all it is a compilation of lived experiences, hopes, fears and possibilities. Zanker and Gard make the astute observation that physical activity can actually "mean different things to one person at the same time" (2008, p. 50). Similarly, for Collier *et al.* (2007) in their study of Irish schoolchildren, sport and physical activity discourses among young people involve *multiple, complex layers*. It is this interplay between the rich and deep range of human involvement and response to physical activity, and the state's various motivations and machinations of activity promotion, that are of interest for this book. I offer here a new definition of physical activity. Physical activity involves people moving, acting and performing within specific spaces and contexts, and influenced by a unique array of interests, emotions, ideas, instructions and relationships.

Clearly then, there is a need to examine the ways in which physical activity is perceived in:

different ways for ...
different groups who live in ...
different places with ...
different motivations for achieving ...
different outcomes.

Interventions that policy makers deploy must be informed not only by good evidence but also by a sympathy for people whose lives are complex and often constrained by unbudgable (and un-nudgable) forces. Being physically active might not only be a healthy thing to do. It might also be deeply political.

Promoting physical activity requires suggesting (and sometimes dictating) what people do with their *time*, their *money*, their *bodies* and their *minds*. By espousing meanings of, reasons for, and policies to promote physical activity, a vast array of experts, from policy makers to academics and health promoters are, without hyperbole, engaged with the meaning of life. Therefore, I move away from a scientific definition of physical activity to account for the inherent social and political nature of all physical activity, acting on and between individuals and communities. For the purposes of this book, I consider physical activity as:

The idea of human movement as a **means** by which an array of political, educational, nationalistic, health, environmental, commercial and personal goals are operationalised, enacted, reinforced and hoped for by institutional and individual bodies.

I emphasise the term 'means' because, for this book, physical activity is a resource which can be deployed in different forms in different spaces by different groups of people. There are three elements to this definition.

- there are various goals,
- there are various ways of achieving them, and
- there are various interest groups.

Thus, physical activity is a very complex political domain. A couple of further points of clarity are offered regarding this definition. First, the emphasis in the definition is not on actual physical activity, but the idea of it. It is the *idea* of movement that is the currency for these organisations. To put this another way, physical activity is rhetorically and discursively constructed well before any person moves. Second, while it is of course the case that regular physical activity can assist with various health markers, this definition aims to disrupt the taken-for-granted 'naturalness' of particular types of physical activity. There is no ideal way to be physically active. Therefore, the ways that are suggested, provided and imposed are of course socially and politically constructed.

Contested histories of physical activities

Organisations that promote physical activities will hold (either explicitly, but more often implicitly) ideas about what physical activities are useful, appropriate or problematic. These ideas are at least partially informed by proclaimed grand truths about physical activity, which have been passed down through the generations, from the ancient world to the present day. Petersson *et al.* (2007) write that "the past is a technology of the present to re-memorialize who 'we' are and have been" (p. 49). In the physical activity policy context this is done through the narrative of 'deficit', that is more people should be doing more activity more often. The 'deficit' narrative makes the past an important feature for two reasons. First, the increasingly invasive measurement of physical activity rates can be automatically compared with those of the recent past, thus repeatedly fuelling policy solutions. Second, and of interest here, are claims and reflections on antiquity. By problematising claims about the past, we might be able to:

- de-romanticise the idea that, in earlier times, people knew the 'true' importance of physical activity and
- de-romanticise the idea that physical activity is unproblematically healthy.

The stories which are told about physical activity have consequences for how current policies are framed. But there is not necessarily anything factual about the stories that are told, especially when stories are told about an ancient past, or more specifically, the *Ancients* who are said to be the storytellers. To show how past understandings about physical activity are borrowed, moulded, shaped and meander over time, Table 2.1 is a timeline about narratives that are employed at different times by different authors in a special issue about physical activity in *The Lancet* medical journal.

Table 2.1 shows how various claims of authors bolster the arguments they are making by choosing narratives that suit their agenda. There is no linearity in the flow of the claims made by the various authors. And so, how do we make sense of these stories? Were the Ancients right about exercise? If so, which ones? Which ones should inform our thinking about physical activity?

Contested futures: what interventions are needed?

To show how these claims can in turn be used to inform policy action of physical activity, Table 2.2 shows how various authors writing about physical activity in *The Lancet* attempt to make claims about the *recent* state of physical activity interventions. As can be seen from the claims below, there is little coherence and much contradiction. However, each claim is used to support the argument of each respective author at a particular moment.

These competing stories pose a problem for establishing a starting point for addressing the issue of inactivity. If much is known about physical activity and many interventions are in place, then any policy action would surely differ vastly from a situation where physical activity has little respect and where interventions are lacking (see Piggin and Bairner, 2014). With this turbulent, often contradictory history and current diagnosis in mind, we can critique the present-day interventions that carry physical activity along as a means by which an array of political, educational, nationalistic, health, environmental, and commercial aims are operationalised, enacted, reinforced and hoped for by a wide array of institutions.

How seriously should we consider physical activity as a matter of public policy? There are two distinct narratives contained within the current discourse. The first is that physical activity is free and/or easy, with

Table 2.1 The transformation of claims about the value of physical activity

Year	Author	Quote
n.d.	Galen of Pergamos	"Athletes live a life quite contrary to the precepts of hygiene, and I regard their mode of living as a regime far more favourable to illness than to health."
1939	Hartley and Llewellyn	[Citing Galen] "The question whether strenuous exercise may lead to strain of the heart and permanent damage to that or other organs, and thus to early death, is one which has excited attention even from the earliest times.... These pronouncements carried great weight, and were, like other Galenic sayings, no doubt accepted as correct throughout the Middle Ages, and, indeed, until much more recent times."
1954	Rook	[Citing Hartley and Llewellyn] "Many observers, both in ancient and in more modern times, have pointed out the alleged dangers of such activities, and these opinions have been summarized by Horton-Smith Hartley and Llewellyn."
2012	Lee *et al.*	[Citing Rook] "Ancient physicians – including those from China in 2600 BC and Hippocrates around 400 BC – believed in the value of physical activity for health. By the 20th century, however, a diametrically opposite view – that exercise was dangerous – prevailed instead."
		"During the early 20th century, complete bed rest was prescribed for patients with acute myocardial infarction."
2012	Wen and Wu	[Citing Lee *et al.*] "Socially, being inactive is perceived as normal, and in fact doctors order patients to remain on bed rest far more often than they encourage exercise."

walking often appearing as both free and easy in physical activity promotion material. The second is that physical activity needs to be thought of as a human right and therefore be elevated on policy agendas (International Sport and Culture Association [ISCA], 2018). (Interestingly, Jeroen Lenaers, a member of the European Parliament from the Netherlands, commented that "I think there should even be a human *duty* to move..."

Table 2.2 Competing claims of physical activity knowledge and action

Page	Authors	Quote
1	Das and Horton (2016)	"The importance of physical activity has been slow to be recognised, and the emphasis to tackle it at a population level has not been forthcoming."
2	Hallal *et al.* (2012)	"For millennia, exercise has been recommended by physicians and scholars. For more than 60 years, science has shown that the health benefits of a physically active lifestyle are extensive and robust."
4	Wen and Wu (2012)	"Exercise … receives little respect from doctors or society … we have few organised efforts to combat physical inactivity." "In addition to doctors' traditional advocacy of the health benefits of exercise …"
45	Heath *et al.* (2012)	"Interventions to increase physical activity in whole populations are now prominent in initiatives, with community-based informational, behavioural, social, policy, and environmental approaches."
76	Kohl *et al.* (2012)	"The role of physical activity continues to be undervalued despite evidence of its protective effects and the cost burden posed by present levels of physical inactivity globally."

(ISCA, 2018, italics added).) One's perspective on this matter will surely affect all that is to follow. Is promotion simply a matter of occasionally encouraging a population to make simple changes, or changing and creating vast arrays of active cultures, policies, environments? If the former, there is no need for the burgeoning number of studies, departments, articles and policy makers who are all interested in the minutiae of activity, from what is the most effective way to walk up stairs for health, to creating best practice guidelines for all manner of target segments. If the latter, if a near fundamental rethink of work practices, funding and communities is needed to turn back the tide of/tackle physical inactivity – this thing which is killing us, then time is of the essence. Whatever the case, given the intensification in physical activity rhetoric in policy domains, it is important to cast a critical eye over policy claims which are laden with particular values over diverse populations. While I wholeheartedly believe that physical activity is good for humans, what inducements and rules are appropriate? What limits should there be on promoting physical activity. How does it shape a populace? In whose interests? The rationales for talking about, researching and intervening in population-wide physical activity extend beyond the state. Corporations and civil society have become very interested in physical activity for various reasons.

Critical approaches to analysing physical activity politics

This book offers various case studies of the state and corporations to examine how, through mechanisms of university research, corporate part-nerships, departments of health, education, transport, et cetera, various organisations have contributed to an intensification and burgeoning of attention on physical activity. What follows is critical analysis. Rather than taking at face value policy decisions and promotional material, the reader will detect the interrogation of stated and hidden aims of physical activity promotion, as well as an examination of the dominant logic that informs it. By asking questions about the motives of those involved in the physical activity industries, we can move towards 'interventions' which are less exploitative, and which result in more positive individual and communal outcomes.

To conduct critical analysis, it is useful to be guided by frameworks sympathetic to the goals of increasing transparency and reducing exploita-tion. To interrogate the machinations of knowledge about physical activity production, this text draws on a range of *critical theories*. Critical theories inform analyses of underlying power struggles and the potential for phys-ical activity to be co-opted by interest groups that have different concerns. Since the policy terrain is inherently political, its analysis must be under-taken with a methodology that acknowledges and accommodates this. It is important to acknowledge that there is no neutral data when it comes to physical activity. Danziger (1995) writes that policy analysis (and ana-lysts) cannot be unbiased: "the potential for professional scientific objec-tivity, political neutrality, or substantive change are, by definition, curtailed significantly ... the givens of any field of activity, are constructed socially and politically" (pp. 436–437). To be clear, I do not argue that facts do not exist, or that there is no truth 'out there'. If someone's pedometer celeb-rates their achievement of 10,000 steps in a day – then I would defer to the supreme measurement capabilities of the device. What is more interesting to me are the political dynamics surrounding the pedometer. Why are they using it? Are they compelled to? How might this influence their perspec-tives about activity? How might evangelical claims about physical activity affect the user? Is there a market involved? Is there a corporation involved? In New Zealand in 2008, McDonalds distributed pedometers to more than 94,000 primary school children who took "three billion steps – walking more than 1.6 million kilometres together and making it the largest physical activity programme ever undertaken in New Zealand" (McDonald's, 2010). There might be more to promoting pedometers than science – there might also be burgers.

Physical activity is a discipline and domain that often relies heavily on the science of health and medical knowledge, possibly to the detriment of other forms of knowledge (Fullagar, 2002; Piggin and Bairner, 2014). Concurrently, there appears to be a paucity of literature on sociology, physical education and sport pedagogy in much physical activity literature. Therefore, *critical theories and approaches* are needed to more fully understand physical activity in populations.

First, adopting a *critical political economy perspective* might help researchers, policy makers and practitioners to reflect on their own unique (and possibly privileged) position about their work. This approach suggests that business can access all levels of decision making and define the political agenda (Blowers, 1983). It emphasises the unequal lobbying and decision-making power inherent in the policy process, unequal resources, and interests which are not always apparent. It is the moments of conflict and contradiction that so often appear in areas of inequality which provide an opportunity to expose unfair practices, faulty logic and allow for interests to be questioned. The approach asks about how we (as citizens and consumers) are encouraged to think about physical activity. How is physical activity being used to alleviate various social ills? How it is being used to ameliorate social injustices? (see Williams *et al.*, 2019). How is physical activity used for exploitative reasons? Who is funding physical activity research and campaigns and whose interests are served by physical activity policies? Of course, it is not just companies which might have a vested interest in the physical activities that its stakeholders partake in. Workplaces, schools, and military establishments all incorporate certain ideas about physical activity into their daily practices. Rather than only trying to promote *more* physical activity, scholars and policy makers alike should critically reflect on the *types* of physical activities that are practised.

Second, *discourse analysis* allows researchers to interrogate the social world of physical activity. Discourse analysis examines how knowledge about a social phenomenon is established, who is interested in maintaining this knowledge, and what the impacts of this knowledge are. For example, discourse analysts might critique interventions which proclaim ideas such as 'anything is possible' or 'be all you can be' for the way they shape people's attitudes towards health. While inspirational slogans might appear unproblematic and inspirational, they might omit the very real constraints of the social milieu. Discourse analysts problematise accepted truths about physical activity, and in turn question the nature of power. One of the most popular writers on discourse is Michel Foucault. He explained that his goal is to "criticize the working of institutions which appear to be both neutral and independent" (Foucault, in Rabinow, 1984, p. 4). Foucault wrote about how power relations are made possible through discourses, and "power must be understood in the first instance as the multiplicity of force relations ... as the process which, through ceaseless struggle and confrontations, transforms, strengthens or reverses [relations of power]" (1978, pp. 92–93). Questions of discipline and freedom are central to Foucault's theories, and are of great importance for physical activity contexts, where judgements are made about the allocation of resources and criteria of inclusion and exclusion into programmes are established (1979a, 1979b, 1980a, 1980b). Also, Foucault's ideas about discourse and power can be applied to both the governance of entire populations and to individual action within institutional settings (Markula and Pringle, 2006; Piggin *et al.*, 2009; Bretherton *et al.*, 2016).

Third, more specifically, a *critical health psychology* (CHP) perspective might be useful for physical activity researchers, policy makers and practitioners. The impetus for a CHP approach is in its political engagement (Murray and Campbell, 2003). CHP 'is concerned with the analysis of social structures and of the social, economic and political issues that produce health, illness, and health care' (Marks, 2004, pp. 79–80). Hepworth (2006) believes various trends are important for health promoters to consider, including aspects of contemporary Western life such as individualism which "reinforces a focus on modifiable 'lifestyle' factors rather than structural determinants of health [and] ... changing relationships between global corporations, governments and affected populations" (Hepworth, 2006, p. 339). For physical activity researchers adopting a critical approach, there is a pressing need to question the political assumptions that are present in all research, which might not be fully apparent. This is not simply an academic exercise. Bernier and Clavier (2011) argue that public health policy researchers should give more attention to politics in order to 'open up unexplored levers of influence' (p. 109). They argue that public health researchers with even a basic literacy in politics and policy.

> would be more likely to question idealistic assumptions about politics and policy-making and be better equipped to get involved in the policy process and enhance their relevance for practitioners and decision-makers dealing with real world problems.
>
> (p. 114)

Critical perspectives acknowledge the potential of physical activity interventions to do *good*, through focus on the unintended (and sometimes intended) problematic, potentially harmful consequences of physical activity policies and practices (see Bercovitz, 2000; Piggin and Lee, 2011).

My approach to applying critical theories to the case studies is intentionally subtle, rather than overbearing. That is to say, the theories and approaches mentioned above inform the analyses which follow, but I also want the case studies to speak for themselves. It was not my intention to over-burden chapters with elongated explanations of the theoretical approaches involved.

Towards less exploitative outcomes

This book is also informed by many writers who discuss the place of the researcher as critic, as researcher and as advocate. Forester (1993) believed that a *critical* approach to analysing public policy can assist in understanding the workings of power. He wrote that this approach can help to see "how policy making and policy implementation reshape the lived worlds of actors [or] restructure social worlds in ways that alter actors' opportunities, capacities to act, and self-conceptions" (p. 12).

Examining the claims made about the physical (in)activity is important, since facts contribute to the allocation of scarce resources and the understanding of possibilities for a population. The way in which these facts are disseminated is also important to consider. For example, in *The Lancet* an evaluation is made of physical education. "The truth is that physical educators have failed ... Physical education itself hasn't delivered physical activity benefits to children in schools" (Khan, in Holmes, 2012, p. 20). Claiming that physical educators have 'failed' might have a potent rhetorical effect. Indeed, it is reasonable to assume that many readers will accept such a remark, particularly since it is framed as 'the truth'. Further, claiming that physical educators have failed serves to delegitimise the profession, allowing other interest groups (such as sport and exercise scientists) to offer solutions to the problem. Blaming (apparently all) physical educators around the world ignores the efforts of physical educators who have taught millions (or billions) of students to understand and use their bodies in healthful ways and spent countless voluntary hours coaching school sports teams. Further, even if physical education was concerned with 'physical activity benefits' in schools, a physical educator might defend their efforts by blaming complex systems, or by citing Stone (2002): "Failures involve so many components and people that it is impossible to attribute blame in any fashion consistent with our cultural norm that responsibility presupposes control" (p. 195). And so less exploitative outcomes come both from changes to material conditions of existence, but also in terms of the respectful allocation of blame for social problems.

What are less exploitative outcomes?

Physical activity promotion imposes specific values on its target population (see Mansfield and Piggin, 2016). To instruct, encourage or compel people to do things with their bodies is inherently political. This is as much the case for technologically advanced, liberal societies as it is for authoritarian, developing economies. The irony for physical activity promoters who value freedom, is that they must necessarily impose ideas, data and measurements on the people they wish to help. Consider terms such as 'intervention' and 'surveillance'. These terms are not value-free or unproblematically good. Who can intervene? What are their motives? Is all surveillance ethical? Can it have unintended, harmful consequences?

'Surveillance' is a term in physical activity promotion that deserves scrutiny. It is a double-edged sword. Populations must be assessed to measure their levels of fitness, but what are the limits of surveillance? When is surveillance inappropriate? When does surveillance, by extending into corporations and schools, become inappropriate? What are the possibilities for people and communities to resist surveillance? Gard (2014) wrote of a looming convergence in electronic health and physical education and asked: "what kind of thing will eHPE be if/when it exists primarily to generate profits and monitor and measure the minutiae of everyday life?" (p. 827). The opportunity to measure, judge, compare one physical activity experience with another might at times be in tension with valuing the freedom of movement, the creativity and the expression that might come from being away from measurement devices.

'Intervention' is a popular tool in physical activity promotion. The term implies an imposition of health onto a population which needs it, whether it knows it or not. Of course, health promoters are most often benevolently concerned about ill health and are eager to make positive change in their communities. Intervening for something as personal and complex as habitual physical activity is a particularly unique policy domain. Able people do at least a little bit of activity, and many people have reasons (or are they excuses!?) for not doing more. The solution is brought to life through the creation of 'physical activity guidelines'. There is regular debate about what types of physical activity need to be promoted. As at the time of writing, there appears to be frustration that strength training is often omitted from physical activity messaging, with the emphasis instead being on aerobic activity (and the implication that cardiovascular fitness is what counts for fitness). Further, there are debates about how to construct persuasive messages –is it a matter of 'every little bit counts'? Or should people assess their activity levels by the day? Or week? (Or hour? Sedentary workers are now often told to not remain sitting for extended periods). Physical activity advocates and promoters are also hindered by relatively free societies – most people cannot be compelled to be physically active (with possible exceptions being prisoners involved in compulsory labour, and school children for whom participation in physical education or sport is compulsory). Most of the population, most of the time, can only be encouraged to be active. Nudged. Enticed. Incentivised. And herein lies the limit of most physical activity interventions. It is difficult to change behaviour of a diverse population, the members of which have unique experiences, preferences and constraints. And so interventions are both value laden and particularly limited in their reach. In this sense, this book parallels Pronger's (2002) attempt to reveal "the ways in which power secrets itself discursively in the seemingly apolitical technology of physical fitness" (p. 11). Beyond the imposition of surveillance and interventions, I offer three examples where outcomes might be challenged or changed in physical activity policy. I hope they serve as examples of how unnecessary or unfair domination might be changed.

Pleasure

In 2002, Brian Pronger wrote about the changes that occurred in his experiences of 'the physical'. He was concerned that the embodied amazement of his active upbringing could not be reconciled with the scientific knowledge of his university training.

> I wrote about 'the powerful source', the wonder and infinity that I discovered in swimming. And I said that when I started to study physical education, that dimension was completely absent from everything we were taught. The technological education I was receiving rendered the wonder second. And as I survey the array of scientific, government and commercial texts on physical fitness, I hear only silence in this regard. The technology of physical [fitness] seems deaf to this dimension of life. So the question of secondness here is: what kind of life is produced in such deafness? But another question also arises: what latent possibilities does that silence hold?
>
> (p. 15)

It is these concerns that inform this text, though they do so in a physical activity sphere that is even more expansive, intensive, commercial and polluted than when Pronger wrote in 2002. Pronger's conceptualisation of "government policies and publications" (p. 126) were confined to "health promotion" and lifestyle management" (p. 126). Pronger does mention healthy communities, healthy and unhealthy cities, and the concepts of ecology and the physical environment, however, he also writes that "the technology of physical fitness does not draw on an ecology of health, focusing instead solely on individual physical and psychology health" (2002, p. 127). This is a distinct point of disjuncture. I argue that the physical activity political discourse now does include into its conception much more of the ecological characteristics than have previously been analysed. We are now far beyond the Canada of 1992 when around "100 internationally recognized experts met to develop consensus on the most important issues through well-prepared preliminary analyses of available information" (Shephard, 1995, p. 288) and concluded that:

> evidence strongly supports the value of regular physical activity in preventing and treating coronary heart disease, hypertension, end-stage renal disease, Type II diabetes mellitus, osteoporosis, certain forms of cancer, surgical trauma, depression, and anxiety. There is also suggestive evidence of benefit in peripheral vascular disease, mild obesity, the chronic phases of rheumatoid and osteoarthritis, and chronic obstructive lung disease …
>
> (Shephard, 1995, p. 288)

While biomedical health still features prominently, other discourses have now become more commonplace, though this is not to say that these other discourses are necessarily liberating or 'healthy'.

To discuss one less exploitative outcome for example, there is certainly space to reconsider pleasure in physical activity promotion. Dallaire *et al.* (2012) found that the recipients of public health messages could in turn create counter-understandings (or reverse discourses) or their experiences of exercise:

> It became clear in some of our interviews that engaging in sport and other physical activities had not been initiated for health reasons, but that the health benefits were a welcome by-product and helped sustain self-regulation. Therefore, the most powerful effects of the fitness discourses in disciplining our participants appear in contexts where physical activity is not only discursively connected to physiological and psychological health, but where it takes on meanings associated with pleasure, sociability and aesthetics.
>
> (p. 336)

Dallaire *et al.* concluded that the "sensation of enjoyment [participants] derived from physical engagement was more powerful in disciplining them into being active than the rationale constructed in health risk discourses" (p. 336). It is also important to note the existence of resistance to dominant ideas about physical activity and health. In Dallaire *et al.*'s (2012) research not-active-enough or inactive participants were unwilling to fully comply with the requirements of the fitness discourses because they found no pleasure in 'exercise'. Further, with regard to pleasure specifically, Phoenix and Orr (2014) argue that pleasure is an under-researched and under-theorised concept within health and health-related areas. Phoenix and Orr

> advocate policy makers and practitioners tasked with promoting regular engagement in physical activity amongst older adults look beyond the 'usual suspects' (e.g., reducing risk of type II diabetes, coronary heart disease, obesity etc.) and bring the notion of pleasure into the foreground of policy making.
>
> (p. 101)

Booth (2009) suggests that the politics of pleasure have resulted in a "prejudice against pleasure in the academy and in state policy" (p. 133). Pronger (2002) also notes that discussions of 'desire' have been limited to questions of (mainly binary homo- and hetero-) sexuality. With this in mind, it is interesting to see that in the latest World Health Organisation global strategy for physical activity (WHO, 2018), the first reference to enjoyment specifically from physical activity appears on page 14, long after the references to risks of heart disease, stroke, diabetes and breast and colon cancer associated with physical inactivity.

Risk

We might also consider the limits of framing physical activity as an unproblematic social good. For instance, boxing, rugby and American football are increasingly being viewed as very risky despite being traditionally lauded for their health benefits. It is reasonable to conclude that young people might be exploited (by being put at risk) for a team's or school's sporting goals. Another example where risk might be considered as a problem is within physically laborious occupations. These can have deleterious consequences for long-term health, and managers around the world might exploit the labour of workers for profit (see Holtermann *et al.*, 2018). That is to say, physical activity is not necessarily synonymous with health.

Uncertainty

Even the 'facts' about physical activity can contradict one another. It appears that the truth about how active a country is depends on who you ask. Population-based measures have grown in prominence, due in part to the increase of surveillance accompanying physical inactivity as a public health issue. An alarmist chart produced by Public Health England in 2014 showed that while the rate of physical inactivity in people aged 15 and over was 18.2 per cent in Holland, it was 63.3 per cent in the UK (Public Health England, 2014, p. 6). Such stark numbers seem intolerable and offer credence to policy actions for urgent change. However, the Global Observatory for Physical Activity (GOPA) claimed somewhat different results. It suggested that the 'prevalence of physical activity' in England in 2012 was 59 per cent for people aged 16 and over (GOPA, 2018), whereas the 'prevalence of physical activity' in the Netherlands in 2013 was very similar at 61 per cent for people aged 18 years and over (GOPA, 2018). Another recent study on child activity levels confirms that vast differences are possible in the reporting of physical activity rates and concludes that "small differences in analysis methods could invalidate cross-country comparisons and at worst will lead to misguided policy and practice" (Williamson *et al.*, 2019, p. 7). Which statistics should we use to inform public policy? Such disparate measures mean we should be wary of statistical claims which provoke unwarranted alarm. This example is also illustrative of the discipline of physical activity being unsettled and contested.

The common rhetoric surrounding physical activity is that interventions need to be both 'evidence-based' and 'innovative'. 'Radical and revolutionary' cultural change is needed and the changes need to be 'industrial scale'. Public Health England (2014) proclaimed that "a pro-activity movement needs to cascade right through society" (p. 12). As critical scholars, we should not take any such proclamations for granted. We should interrogate them, unpack them and test their logic. It is the hidden and possibly unaccounted-for dynamics of construction that are of interest here. It is not the goal to construct a perfect, coherent story about the history and meaning of physical activity. Rather, by illuminating inaccuracies, misrepresentations and over-reaches we might first encourage scepticism about grand proclamations, and second, open space to develop a critical and ethical approach to physical activity promotion. And so, armed with an array of approaches to apply to the domain of physical activity, the following chapters aim to educate, provoke and advance thinking about physical activity politics.

22 *Contested definitions, histories, futures*

References

Bercovitz, K. (2000). A critical analysis of Canada's 'Active Living': Science or politics? *Critical Public Health, 10*(1), 19–39.

Bernier, N.F. and Clavier, C. (2011). Public health policy research: Making the case for a political science approach. *Health Promotion International, 26*(1), 109–116.

Biddle, S.J.H. and Mutrie, N. (2001). *Psychology of Physical Activity: Determinants, Well-being and Interventions.* London: Routledge.

Blowers, A. (1983). Master of fate or victim of circumstance: The exercise of corporate power in environmental policy-making. *Policy and Politics, 11*, 393–415.

Booth, D. (2009). Politics and pleasure: The philosophy of physical education revisited. *Quest, 61*(2), 133–153.

Bretherton, P., Piggin, J. and Bodet, G. (2016). Olympic sport and physical activity promotion: The rise and fall of the London 2012 pre-event mass participation 'legacy'. *International Journal of Sport Policy and Politics, 8*(4), 609–624.

Bull, F.C. and Bauman, A.E. (2011). Physical inactivity: The 'Cinderella' risk factor for noncommunicable disease prevention. *Journal of Health Communication: International Perspectives*, 16(sup2), 13–26.

Collier, C., MacPhail, A. and O'Sullivan, M. (2007). Student discourse on physical activity and sport among Irish young people. *Irish Educational Studies, 26*(2), 195–210.

Dallaire, C., Lemyre, L., Krewski, D. and Gibbs, L.B. (2012). The gap between knowing and doing: How Canadians understand physical activity as a health risk management strategy. *Sociology of Sport Journal, 29*(3), 325–347.

Danziger, M. (1995). Policy analysis postmodernized. *Policy Studies Journal, 23*(3), 435–450.

Das, P. and Horton, R. (2016). Physical activity: Time to take it seriously and regularly. *The Lancet*, 388, 1254–1255.

Forester, J. (1993). *Critical Theory, Public Policy and Planning Practice: Towards a Critical Pragmatism.* Albany: State University of New York Press.

Foucault, M. (1978). *The History of Sexuality, Volume 1: The Will to Knowledge.* London: Penguin.

Foucault, M. (1979a). *Discipline and Punish: The Birth of the Prison.* UK. Harmondsworth.

Foucault, M. (1979b). Governmentality. *Ideology and Consciousness, 6*, 5–21.

Foucault, M. (1980a). Prison talk. In C. Gordon (ed.), *Power/Knowledge: Selected Interviews and Other Writings 1972–1977*, (pp. 55–62). Harlow, England: Harvester.

Foucault, M. (1980b). Body/Power. In C. Gordon (ed.), *Power/knowledge: Selected Interviews and Other Writings 1972–1977* (pp. 55–62). Harlow, England: Harvester.

Fullagar, S. (2002). Governing the healthy body: Discourses of leisure and lifestyle within Australian health policy. *Health, 6*(1), 69–84.

Gard, M. (2014). eHPE: A history of the future. *Sport, Education and Society, 19*(6), 827–845.

GOPA (2018). Country cards. Retrieved from www.globalphysicalactivity observatory.com/

Hallal, P.C., Bauman, A.E., Heath, G.W., Kohl, H.W., Lee, I. and Pratt, M. (2012). Physical activity: More of the same is not enough. *The Lancet, 380*(9838), 190–191.

Hartley, P.H.-S. and Llewellyn, G.F. (1939). An investigation into the longevity of Cambridge sportsmen. *British Medical Journal, 1*, 657.

Heath, G.W., Parra, D.C., Sarmiento, O.L., Andersen, L.B., Owen, N., Goenka, S., Montes, F. and Brownson, R.C. (2012). Evidence-based intervention in physical activity: Lessons from around the world. *The Lancet, 380*(9838), 272–281.

Hepworth, J. (2006). The emergence of critical health psychology: Can it contribute to promoting public health? *Journal of Health Psychology, 11*(3), 331–341.

Holmes, D. (2012). Profile: Karim Khan: Good sport. *The Lancet, 380*(9836), 20.

Holtermann, A., Krause, N., van der Beek, A.J. and Straker, L. (2018). The physical activity paradox. *British Journal of Sports Medicine, 52*, 149–150.

International Sport and Culture Association [ISCA] (2018). Everybody should have the Human Right to MOVE and play: MEPs share their views. Retrieved from www.youtube.com/watch?v=pLLhhQmv4Eo

Kohl, H.W., Craig, C.L., Lambert, E.V., Inoue, S., Alkandari, J.R., Leetongin, G. and Kahlmeier, S., for the Lancet Physical Activity Series Working Group (2012). The pandemic of physical inactivity: Global action for public health. *The Lancet, 380*(9838), 294–305.

Lee, I.-M., Shiroma, E.J., Lobelo, F., Puska, P., Blair, S.N. and Katzmarzyk, P.T., for the Lancet Physical Activity Series Working Group (2012). Effect of physical inactivity on major noncommunicable diseases worldwide: An analysis of burden of disease and life expectancy. *The Lancet, 380*(9838), 219–229.

Mansfield, L. and Piggin, J. (2016). Sport, physical activity and public health. *International Journal of Sport Policy and Politics, 8*(4), 533–537.

Marks, D.F. (2004). Rights to health, freedom from illness: A life and death matter. In M. Murray (ed.), *Critical Health Psychology* (pp. 61–82). London: Palgrave.

Markula, P. and Pringle, R. (2006). *Foucault, Sport and Exercise: Power, Knowledge and Transforming the Self.* New York: Routledge.

McDonald's (2010). 100,000 Kiwi kids stride towards FIFA World Cup. Retrieved from https://mcdonalds.co.nz/sites/mcdonalds.co.nz/files/100000_kiwi_kids_stride_towards_fifa_world_cup_media.pdf

Milton, K. and Bauman, A. (2015). A critical analysis of the cycles of physical activity policy in England. *International Journal of Behavioral Nutrition and Physical Activity, 12*(1), Article 8.

Murray, M. and Campbell, C. (2003). Beyond the sidelines: Towards a more politically engaged health psychology. *Health Psychology Update, 12*(3), 12–17.

Petersson, K., Olsson, U. and Popkewitz, T. (2007). Nostalgia, the future, and the past as pedagogical technologies. *Discourse: Studies in the Cultural Politics of Education, 28*(1), 49–67.

Phoenix, C. and Orr, N. (2014). Pleasure: A forgotten dimension of physical activity in older age. *Social Science and Medicine, 115*, 94e102.

Piggin, J. and Bairner, A. (2014). The global physical inactivity pandemic: An analysis of knowledge production. *Sport, Education and Society, 21*(2), 131–147.

Piggin, J., Jackson, S. and Lewis, M. (2009). Knowledge, power and politics: Contesting 'evidence-based' national sport policy. *International Review for the Sociology of Sport, 44*, 87–101.

Piggin, J. and Lee, J. (2011). 'Don't mention obesity': Contradictions and tensions in the UK Change4Life health promotion campaign. *Journal of Health Psychology, 16*, 1151–1164.

Pronger, B. (2002). *Body Fascism: Salvation in the Technology of Physical Fitness.* Toronto: University of Toronto Press.

Public Health England (2014). *Everybody Active, Every Day: An Evidence-based Approach to Physical Activity.* London: Public Health England.

Rabinow, P. (ed.) (1984). *The Foucault Reader: An Introduction to Foucault's Thoughts and other Writings 1972–1977.* Harlow, England: Harvester Press.

Rook, A. (1954). An investigation into the longevity of Cambridge sportsmen. *British Medical Journal, 1*, 773–777.

Shephard, R.J. (1995). Physical activity, fitness, and health: The current consensus. *Quest, 47*(3), 288–303.

Stone, D. (2002). *Policy Paradox: The Art of Political Decision Making.* New York: W.W. Norton.

Wen, C.P. and Wu, X. (2012). Stressing harms of physical inactivity to promote exercise. *The Lancet, 380*(9838), 192–193.

Williams, O., Coen, S.E. and Gibson, K. (2019). Comment on: 'Equity in Physical Activity: A Misguided Goal'. *Sports Medicine.* doi: doi.org/10.1007/s40279-018-01047-9

WHO (2017). Health topics: Physical activity. Retrieved from www.who.int/topics/physical_activity/en/

WHO (2018). *Global Action Plan on Physical Activity 2018–2030: More Active People for a Healthier World.* Geneva: World Health Organisation.

Williamson, C., Kelly, P. and Strain, T. (2019). Different analysis methods of Scottish and English child physical activity data explain the majority of the difference between the national prevalence estimates. *BMC Public Health.* doi: doi.org/10.1186/s12889-019-6517-7

Zanker, C. and Gard, M. (2008). Fatness, fitness, and the moral universe of sport and physical activity. *Sociology of Sport Journal, 25*(1), 48–65.

3 Towards a physical activity discourse

This chapter has two objectives. First, to present a model of the political discourse of physical activity. Second, to explain the ways in which the discourse manifests itself in the polity (in organised society).

What is physical activity in academia and policy? Is it a field? A discipline? A sub-discipline? Is it a type of medicine? Perhaps it is some of the above, but I would argue that more importantly, in the policy realm it has developed into a specific *political discourse*. Discourses are powerful because they actively produce what we know. Discourses govern the way a topic can be meaningfully talked about, reasoned about, as well as influencing how ideas are put into practice and used to regulate the conduct of others. Just as a discourse 'rules in' certain ways of talking about a topic, defining an acceptable and intelligible way to talk, write and conduct oneself, it also rules out, limits and restricts other ways of talking and conducting oneself (Hall, 1997).

It is not enough to simply accept the rationalities that physical activity interest groups and promoters offer as the totality of understanding of physical activity. Instead we should examine what is assumed in policy proclamations, what is subtle, and what is purposefully unwritten or omitted. This is particularly the case since physical activity lobbyists appear to be evoking and eliciting a wide variety of benefits that come from physical activity. For example, it is referred to as medicine, a magic pill, a golden thread, among other metaphors.

To analyse the emergence of a discourse about physical activity at a political/policy level, I am guided broadly by Foucault's archaeological analysis (1972). Foucault argued that discourses within society change over time, and he wanted to identify the birth and growth of discourses and the conditions which gave impetus to them. Discourse change might occur at times when "the scales or guidelines have been displaced ... the information system has been modified ... [and] the lexicon of signs and their decipherment has been entirely reconstituted" (1972, p. 37).

Foucault noted that it is not easy to say something 'new'. New discourses become established when the conditions "are many and imposing ... under the positive conditions of a complex group of relations" (p. 49). Also imperative are relations between institutions, economic and social processes, behavioural patterns and systems of norms, as well as a discursive system of relations that enables a discourse to appear. It is these discursive relations that "offer a discourse objects of which it can speak" (p. 51). Ultimately, Foucault hoped to show that "in analysing discourses themselves, one sees the loosening of the embrace, apparently so tight, of words and things, and the emergence of a group of rules proper to discursive practice" (p. 54). An archaeological investigation aimed to show how "ideas could appear, sciences be established, experience be reflected in philosophies, rationalities be formed ..." (1970, xxii). Foucault (1972) argued that an archaeology should show "how the prohibitions, exclusions, limitations, values, freedoms, and transgressions ... all its manifestations, verbal or otherwise, are linked to a discursive practice" (p. 213). As such, any archaeological, discursive analysis must take into consideration what is excluded (or marginalised) from mainstream policy discourse.

Some attention has been paid to the discursive machinations of the health-fitness nexus specifically. Markula and Pringle (2006) wrote about how Foucault's archaeological approach could be deployed in the area of sport and exercise. To distinguish, Markula and Pringle emphasise analysis on workings of power on individual bodies, whereas I emphasise the political and policy machinations of the workings of discourses. However, there is overlap here. Whether fitness or physical activity, Markula and Pringle emphasise the need to examine objects, enunciations, concepts and theories about the subject of study:

- The objects of physical activity include and extend beyond the body, to the environment, the company, the school, etc.
- The enunciations include the media and sites in which the objects appear. These appear in government reports, in policy documents, in ad campaigns and so on.
- Concepts include the justifications for the discourse, such as health, education, sustainability, notions of social capital development, social cohesion and so on. Later I refer to these as an interplay between sustaining discourses and interest themes.
- Theories, those "regulated ways of practicing the possibilities of discourse" (Foucault, 1972, p. 64) will involve those ways of solving/ addressing the physical activity problem based on the concept mentioned above. At a policy/political level, this will involve choices

about resource distribution, the authorising of certain groups to represent the problem, ideas about 'scaling up', including 'everyone' and so on.

Rather than a scientific discipline, Markula and Pringle refer to fitness as a "coherent discursive formation" (p. 53). This definition could also be applied to physical activity. While there is overlap between 'fitness' and physical activity, I proceed on the basis of some distinctions too, as physical activity is extending its discursive tentacles into numerous other political spheres and disciplines, as will be discussed later in this chapter. Nevertheless, Markula and Pringle note that the concepts "physical activity, fitness and health appear to form a 'group relation' that allows for further theoretical formulations" regarding what it means to have a physically fit body (p. 56). This analysis deals mainly with discourse at a political/policy level and, as such, 'policy archaeology' is used (Scheurich, 1994, 1997). Following Scheurich's explanation, this political/policy archaeology is guided by four themes. These include

1 an analysis of the social construction of the problem,
2 how policy choices are shaped by social regularities,
3 an examination of a discourse's ability to define solutions,
4 an analysis of the legitimatisation process and effect of the new discourse.

It is important to delineate the powerful cultural, political and economic forces which have and are informing our understandings of physical activity. In the past two decades, there has been an expansion and intensification of interventions to produce more physically active populations. In order to map the emergence of this new physical activity discourse, it is necessary to step back from the compartmentalised view of the domain which often dominates our thinking and consider what forces, connections and elements have contributed to bring about the current vital (life or death) burden which is imposed upon human movement. Later, a framework is proposed to show how the physical activity discourse has come about. Before a detailed examination of the framework, it is necessary to make some general remarks about the preconditions of the framework.

The physical activity discourse, I argue here, has not emerged from nowhere. Other discourses, like antecedent ingredients, have facilitated the escalation in physical activity's rise to prominence and legitimacy. These include the *obesity epidemic* which has framed human bodies as susceptible to judgement and surveillance (see Gard and Wright, 2005).

Physical education's struggle for disciplinary legitimacy over decades has not resulted in a specialism that can/would/should govern the physical health of young human bodies in many countries. The rise of *surveillance technologies* which affect both leisure and work domains (see Lupton, 2012) has allowed physical activity to be measured ad infinitum (and ad nauseum). Continued socio-economic inequalities, increasingly intense urbanisation (with associated environment degradation), and post-industrial (sedentary) labour forces have also been underlying factors in the rise of physical activity to prominence as a major health issue.

Of course, the discourse does not still appear with all these ingredients. It needs a raft of committed 'bakers' who will devote time and attention to escalate and seek legitimacy for physical activity. Networks are needed, most obviously manifesting as scientific associations of physical activity. And with these scholarly societies come links to industry and the state. (Indeed, the state–academic–commercial nexus of physical activity is worthy of specific discussion later). And so, there is no particular origin of the physical activity discourse. Instead, after scientific elements establish legitimacy, it is continually built upon and deployed in different spheres, with frontiers in all directions. Indeed, this framework for thinking about the physical activity discourse is not intended to be static. There will be specific contexts which frame physical activity in unique ways. That is part of what makes the discourse a potentially powerful policy driver. Its hybridity and its potential omnipresence as a matter of concern (affecting all domains of human life) means that it can be potentially infused into all sorts of policies.

Before offering the theory of the physical activity political discourse, it is necessary to say something of theory building. Shoemaker *et al.* (2003) write that

> theory building is difficult because it requires both great discipline and great creativity, and although a person may possess one of these attributes, few people seem to possess both.... It requires both excruciating attention to detail coupled with wild flights of imagination.
>
> (p. 10)

The model in Figure 3.1 has not been produced from a focus on one source, but through evaluation and reflection during a continuing career, having worked in university Schools of Physical Education, and Exercise and Health, and taught in the disciplines of management, policy sciences, marketing, and in the melting pot of 'health sciences'. My research over the last 15 years has focused on power relations within state and corporate organisations and their attempts to produce more active people. And so

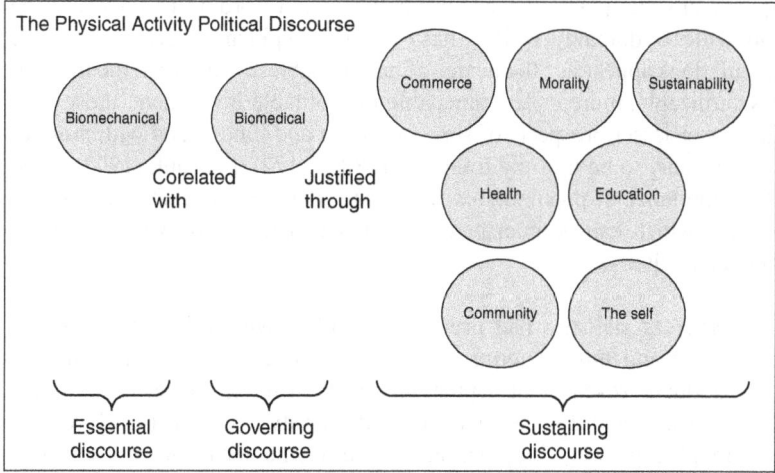

Figure 3.1 The physical activity political discourse model.

this model is the first attempt (after many drafts) to elucidate and explicate the current political discourse of physical activity.

This discourse presented here informs the polity, which here is taken to include the state–academic–commercial nexus. The elements of the discourse are discussed below.

Essential discourse: biomechanics

At the core of the physical activity discourse is biomechanics. The goal of biomechanics is to measure human movement. Humans moving in one place, or from one place to another, repeatedly, over time is the core of the discipline around which everything else hangs. While I suggest it is an essential discourse, it does not carry a great amount of disciplinary weight when the topic is researched, analysed or justified. Human movement without values added is not enough to produce and sustain the physical activity discourse. Biomechanical data without value is inanimate. It must be animated (or brought to life) by one or more rationalities. Justifications for movement are needed. It is not enough by itself.

Governing discourse: biomedical

Undoubtedly, the biomedical domain made connections between physical activity, health and death rates. It is useful here to contextualise more widely the powerful connection between statistics and populations and specifically the place of medical knowledge. According to Foucault, the biomedical domain which has allowed epidemiologists to make populations appear as "the bearer of new variables ... between the more or less utilizable, more or less amenable to profitable investment, those with greater or lesser prospects of survival, death and illness, and with more or less capacity to be usefully trained" (1980, p. 172). Foucault (1994) noted the importance of population-wide data for the identification of aspects of society which can be managed or changed, particularly with relation to death and disease:

> Whereas statistics had previously worked within the administrative frame and thus in terms of the functioning of sovereignty, it now gradually reveals that population has its own regularities, its own rate of deaths and diseases, its cycles of scarcity, etc; statistics show also that the domain of population involves phenomena that are irreducible to those of the family, such as epidemics, endemic levels of mortality, ascending spirals of labour and wealth...
>
> (p. 218)

Most often individuals do not connect their physical activity levels with imminent death. However, by aggregating population-wide data, epidemiologists have been able to connect physical activity over time with premature death. It is this linkage which has allowed the importance of physical activity to be framed as an essential matter for public policy. This has led to physical activity being elevated quickly up the list of measurable behaviours which individuals are obliged to monitor, measure and change if needed, which medical personnel are required to consult patients on, and which researchers are bound to measure and attempt to change through interventions.

The biomedical discourse has not just allowed the physical activity discourse to be created. It also justifies physical activity in an ongoing sense, with longitudinal surveillance over time used to measure the effects of interventions. While there are other discourses which inform the physical activity discourse, it is the biomedical discourse which justifies physical activity as a vital sphere to continually treat as a matter on ongoing concern and intervene in. However, to do so, various sustaining discourses, or proxies are deployed too. What becomes apparent from the literature (academic, policy and commercial) is that the specific reasons for moving become secondary to the benefits that come from it. A biomechanical foundation is used as the basis around which all the other rationalities, motivations and logics flow.

Sustaining discourses

Commerce

Tying any social problem to commercial imperatives is as common as it is problematic. Individuals' quests for health, anti-ageing/youth, beauty, fitness and vitality are well understood as being appealing for consumers and lucrative for companies. While commerce is not an obvious discourse to sustain physical activity, it does so in two ways. First, a proxy for commerce is the utilisation of the 'economy' (which assumes costs to the economy is negative). In 2016 a *Lancet* article claimed "in addition to morbidity and premature mortality, physical inactivity is responsible for a substantial economic burden" (Ding *et al.*, 2016 p. 1311) The authors suggest "the total economic burden of physical inactivity in 2013 was estimated to range from $67·5 billion (18·5–182·1) in a conservative analysis to $145·2 billion (47·0–338·8) in a less conservative analysis" (p. 1322). These data certainly appear alarming and contribute another previously uncounted aspect of the problem of physical inactivity.

The second way in which commerce is evoked is subtler. The profit incentives of corporations have long informed how companies are obliged interact with their customers. In recent years, two companies have been at the forefront of physical activity promotion – Nike and Coca Cola. Both companies in different ways have sought to integrate themselves into the physical activity community in order to generate profit. Both companies could simply be viewed as connecting ideas and markets for profit (as indeed they are legally obligated to do). However, when considered in connection with ideas about public health (another important discourse in physical activity promotion), then these efforts can be seen to be problematic.

One powerful example of the attempted influence of industry comes from Coca Cola and the defunct Global Energy Balance Network (GEBN). The GEBN ostensibly advocated for physical activity, but allegations surfaced of attempts to conceal the private and vested interests in its endeavour, to the extent that it was accused of downplaying the significance of diet as a factor in health conditions such as obesity, and placing the blame on physical inactivity instead. This partnership between university researchers and corporate interests of the Coca Cola Company drew significant and wide-ranging public criticism, and the 'Network' would eventually close (O'Connor, 2015).

Morality

Morality in this context refers to the idea that participation in physical activity is 'good' not just for the individual, but for society in general. Its relative goodness relates to other discourses, such as environmental sustainability and tax payer savings. This idea is infused throughout, and is a key component of, physical activity promotions. We can see this discourse present in many contexts, from the appeal to personal responsibility for physical activity claims which mention how easy it is to participate, to the connection with decreasing public health care costs. In this way, the active citizen (as connoted by an absence of body fat or presence at physical activity events) is doing their part for health.

Appeals to 'ancient' knowledge are also deployed in physical activity rhetoric, with academics reaching back to Greek or Chinese texts to show the reader that physical activity is *virtuous* (Lee *et al.*, 2012). Dallaire *et al.* (2012) also discuss physical activity as being imbued with morality. They argue that in many neo-liberal states, "a physically active lifestyle is discursively constructed as a moral activity, whereas a sedentary lifestyle is criticized and viewed as a failure to take charge of one's health" (p. 326). Zanker and Gard (2008) highlight how morality is infused into the physical activity discourse through its connection with the obesity epidemic. They argue that current scientific and popular discussions of obesity and physical activity are morally loaded so that, for example, being classified as overweight or obese is seen as a personal moral failing. Indeed, with international comparisons increasingly available, results can be used to lament, and subsequently blame people or policy for 'failing' to live up to guidelines imposed by the physically activity community. Interestingly, Zanker and Gard (2008) argue that

> By presenting physical activity to young people as a kind of insurance against all the bad things that could go wrong in their lives, we lie to them, both in terms of the scientific evidence on health and physical activity and in loading physical activity with spurious moral weight.
>
> (p. 64)

Health

Related to, yet also distinct from the biomedical discourse, is the healthism discourse, which manifests as populations being directed to be concerned about their own health. For Fitzpatrick and Tinning (2014), notions of healthism refer to the desire to improve health and the subsequent drive for "many people to monitor their bodies and stems from a concern for being healthy, eating healthily and behaving in health-enhancing way" (p. 5). The health discourse is the most apparent in the physical activity sphere. Dallaire *et al.* (2012) note that various health organisations offer "expert discursive fragments", whereby physical activity becomes medicalised and is prescribed (in Canada) to promote a culture where individuals are responsible for their well-being. This echoes Pronger (2002), who argued that "the governments of most industrial and post-industrial countries now actively promote programs and support scientific research to develop the fitness of their populations" (p. 3). Health is of course intimately connected with all aspects of daily life, the tasks focused on, the air breathed, the food eaten, the jobs undertaken, and the community one is connected with can all be evaluated in terms of how healthy or unhealthy they are. It seems there is no escape from health concerns. Physical activity, with its place at the intersection of so many measurable factors, is thus at the epicentre of health concerns. A 2009 editorial in the *British Journal of Sports Medicine* opined that physical inactivity is "the biggest public health problem of the 21st century" (Blair, 2009). This was certainly an overly grandiloquent claim. Aside from the apparent exclusion of poverty, political instability and climate change as contenders for biggest public health problem, it is possible that there are other challengers for this title. However, such a claim does have a powerful rhetorical effect. It focuses the mind on something that seems both pertinent and changeable. The importance of measures of physical fitness, mental health, longevity, DALYs (Disability Adjusted Life Years), step counts, calories and so on all feed into a focus on an individual's health and help shape solutions. If we can measure a problem, we can intervene and solve it.

Dallaire *et al.* (2012) note that physical activity is one such method promoted as an effective means of managing health risks and, therefore, of controlling citizens' bodies. Pronger (2002) describes the technology of physical fitness as a discourse of texts, sociocultural practices, and bodily procedures that produce human life in controlled ways:

> increased physical control in terms of muscular strength, endurance, and flexibility, and greater cardio-vascular efficiency for the sake of better athletic performance or greater control over health in terms of disease prevention, both physical and mental living longer and more efficiently, for instance.... [It] also plays a growing role in sculpting the body for a fashionable look, typically, lean, muscular and youthful.
>
> (p. xiv)

Pronger and a number of critical educational scholars examine the particularly problematic aims and effects of healthism, from teaching young people "to manage their own relationship with and to the risks of the environment, which are seen to be everywhere and in everything" (Petersen and Lupton, 1996, p. xi), to the imposition of body ideals.

Sustainability

Connected to this idea of health is the discourse of sustainability, which has increased in a variety of politico-economic spheres in recent decades (Christen and Schmidt, 2012). The recent adoption of systems thinking and 'ecological approaches' situates physical activity not just as something to be done for personal health reasons, but for its effects on the environment. There is a synergy between these ideas. Active transport features prominently in connecting movement with both the environment and environmentalism. Cyclists, for example, are not only active the world, but are polluting it less than a stereotypical motorist would. The dominant logics of sustainable activity are that sedentary behaviours and technologies related to passive consumption should be problematised, and that 'radical' thinking might be needed to instigate significant change. Active transport, bike lanes, green technology and public transport are perceived to be the major levers to create change. Indeed, this appears to be one of the most potent discourses for physical activity today, with awareness of environmental damage, emerging green technologies, increasing awareness of the physical harms of pollution, and increasingly mobile (but not active) populations.

Education

When discussing education, it is the primary and secondary school systems that are the default sites for physical activity interventions. They are also the places where a population is most often targeted for interventions. Physical education in many countries faces ongoing struggles over its place in school curricula, whether it is through perceived legitimacy, conflict with crammed timetables, a lack of resources, a prioritisation of or conflation with competitive sport, and perceived increasingly sedentary behaviours of young people (see Gard and Vander Schee, 2014). This ties into the emphasis on 'health' – whereby physical education has always been associated with the medical discourse of health (see Tinning, 2010; Jung et al., 2016). In recent years the concept of physical literacy has gained prominence as a frame of reference for the benefits that come from knowledge and competence around particular ways of moving (see Edwards et al., 2017).

Physical education is not just in the remits of formal education systems. Pronger (2002) notes that physical fitness has become the centrepiece of physical education for children, adults and the elderly, and further, scientific knowledge and the scientisation of physical education have been centred in the production of social control. Pronger (2002) attempted to reveal "the ways in which power secrets itself discursively in the seemingly apolitical technology of physical fitness" (p. 11). It is certainly the case that both formal and informal education settings are imbued with a wide variety of learning pedagogies – hopes and opportunities to be taught and learn new skills and ways of being. Of course, many of these are positive, and enable the recipient to be more free, creative and expressive. It is also certainly the case though, that there are other dominant, desired objectives and commercial interests at play in this domain.

Community

Appeals to community spirit, community development, community cohesion are core aspects of modern policy justifications for promoting physical activity. Consider this framing by Das and Horton regarding the physical inactivity pandemic:

> This Series on physical activity is not about sport and it is about more than just exercise. It is about the relationship between human beings and their environment, and about improving human wellbeing by strengthening that relationship. *It is not about running on a treadmill, whilst staring at a mirror and listening to your iPod...*
>
> (Das and Horton, 2012, p. 1, italics added)

In this case physical activity is framed as artificial (the treadmill), narcissistic (staring at a mirror) and antisocial (the iPod). Notwithstanding the fact there are other interpretations of such behaviour (as safe, time out from a stressful life), the idea of social interaction through physical activity is a desired way of organising. The World Health Organisation emphasises community as a core part in its mission, using physical activity "as a means of improving individual and community health..." (WHO, 2018a, p. 8). Community settings are of course where the practical interventions into people's lives must take place, whether it is through inspirational mass media campaigns or council-led fitness classes, the idea of getting community 'buy-in' to interventions through consultation and co-creation is also becoming more prominent within the physical activity promotion milieu.

Connected with the discourse of community are ideas of inclusion and diversity. For many years, these terms have been unproblematic, positive, feel-good, 'up' words, though in recent times, broader political shifts towards populism and nationalism might be destabilising these ideals. In the UK, when Prime Minister Theresa May, wrote that "We will take back control of our borders, by putting an end to the free movement of people once and for all" (May, 2018), it indicated a desire to exclude, in some sense, others.

The self

The idea of physical activity contributing to a person's well-being is not new. The discourse of the self – as it relates to physical activity – is popular and expressed in numerous ways. 'Attaining' health, well-being, fulfilment, self-actualisation, are all connected with being in some type of control over the body and how it is used. In the policy sphere, this discourse is becoming more prominent, and there are many parallels between it and neo-liberal thinking about health promotion, the ideas that the individual is ultimately responsible for their own health (connecting with the health discourse above). A critical perspective would hold that some health promotions would work to reinforce "discourses of self-regulation as good citizenship" (Smith Maguire, 2002). It is also apparent though, that with the appreciation of entrenched social structures and their effect on life chances (including physical health), that the creation of the self occurs within a system of constraints and broader social processes. And so there is an interplay between discourses of blame for ill health, inspirational health promotion campaigns, and behind-the-scenes policy levers which attempt to alter life chances of those not deemed to be physically active enough.

The political discourse model with interest frames included

An expanded model (Figure 3.2) is also offered to account for examples of the wide variety of 'interest frames' that inform thinking about physical activity from a political perspective. It is likely that most of the sustaining discourses of physical activity are informed by interest groups and populations with unique values. These dominant interest frames – Culture, Gender, Age, Dis/ability, Ethnicity, Religion, Material wealth and Developmental state – are limited here for concision. It is likely there are many more interest frames which interact with the sustaining discourses at different times. The two-way arrow conveys that while these interest frames influence the utilisation of physical activity discourses, these discourses might also contribute to the identities of various interest groups.

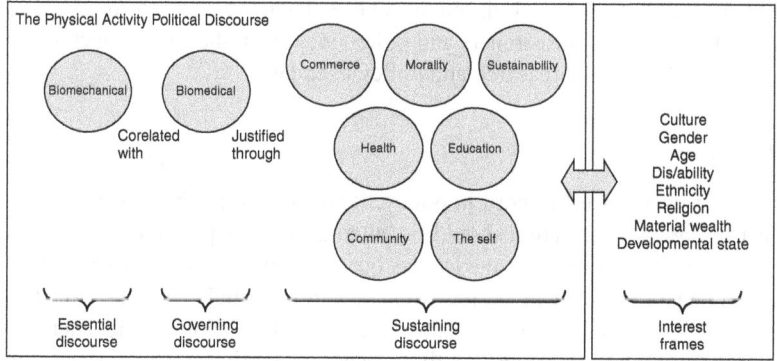

Figure 3.2 The physical activity political discourse model with interest frames included.

The proposed way in which these interest frames are utilised is by way of a simplified case study of gender. Many states conduct surveillance on the two traditionally dominant gender categories, and increasingly account for an expanded conception of gender. The result of these measures leads to targeted promotional campaigns for a gendered target market to do more physical activity. (Of course, there are intersectional aspects at play, with campaigns accounting for more than gender.) With the targeting of a gender, the activity promoters choose from one or more sustaining discourses to define what physical activity is about for the targeted gender. It may promote activity for a woman's *self*-confidence, it might appeal to a developing *sense of community*, and or it might emphasise *commercial* imperatives of saving money through active transport, which in turn utilises a *sustainability* discourse. In turn, these values might reinforce perceptions of the interest frames.

The characteristics of the physical activity discourse

As mentioned at the start of this chapter, the polity in this case represents the totality of institutions involved in the production and sustenance of the physical activity discourse. This will include universities, the formal state machinery (from its expert groups to committees to health bodies), the schooling system (both public and private), and the corporate sphere, with its legal and insatiable goal of generating profit. Managers within these institutions will choose how to deploy sustaining discourses and interest frames for their own members or target market, as the multidimensional nature of the discourse allows for flexibility in its use.

This following section highlights a range of dominant themes within the physical activity political discourse. These characteristics inform physical activity promoters, researchers and policy makers in their pronouncements and contribute to the research and policy agendas.

Urgency

Urgency is a powerful word in policy. It suggests something is more than just important, that action should be taken as soon as possible to change a detrimental situation. This device has become ubiquitous in both advocacy campaigns for physical activity and scientific article conclusions. For example, Guthold *et al.* (2018) concluded that "Policies to increase population levels of physical activity need to be prioritised and scaled up urgently" (p. e1077). The UK All Party Commission on Physical Activity (2014) claimed "We need urgent action to reverse this trend" (p. 3). Hallal *et al.* (2012) stated "technological advancements that nudge us towards physical inactivity make it urgently necessary to take actions" (p. 190). These are only a few examples of a sentiment which pervades calls to action. The limitation with calls for urgency, like other slow-moving problems (such as global warming, poverty or obesity), is that because of the often (potential) temporally distal negative consequences, a sense of urgency is difficult to sustain unless advocacy is constant and well-targeted.

Totality

Connected with earlier discussions about the variety of other discourses that contribute to physical activity, it is apparent that the problem of inactivity is increasingly framed as manifesting in every place, for everyone, every day. A claim is made in *The Lancet* that a "*complete understanding* of all stakeholders, their interactions, and how their interactions make up the whole is crucial to understanding of the systems that impede progress on physical activity" (Kohl *et al.*, p. 302, italics added). All people can be targeted. All urban and rural settings can be targeted. Of course, this is an immensely benevolent sentiment, though it might also be overbearing when every sedentary act is reframed into a potentially risky behaviour (even sitting!). This totality is brought into existence in part by technologies of surveillance, such as pedometers and accelerometers which allow human movement over an entire 24 hours to be monitored. It intensifies ideas about risk in all settings, such as sitting in workplaces and schools. However, this rhetorical device is most apparent in optimistic policy names, such as Public Health England's

(2014) 'Everybody Active, Every Day'. This is hyperbolic, but when such rhetoric gains legitimacy through formal policy pronouncements, it brings all activities under the umbrella of legitimate scrutiny and surveillance. Consider too the framing of physical activity in the UK Government's long-term health campaign. The UK Change4Life literature included the justification that the campaign was needed because:

> Change4Life is a society-wide movement that encourages everyone to make changes to their diet and activity levels in order to reverse the growing trend of obesity and obesity related illnesses. At the broadest level, our target audience is everyone in England, as everyone is potentially at risk.
>
> (DOH, 2009, p. 5)

Such a claim would mean that no one in the UK is as healthy as they should be. Through this totality comes the related idea of complexity, and the subsequent systems approaches which must be deployed to understand complexity.

Global

The discourse of the global nature of the problem is now entrenched into academic parlance. The framing of the issue as a 'global' pandemic by the authors of the 2012 *Lancet* special issue on physical activity legitimised the far geographical reach and the subsequent need to intervene in communities around the world. The differentiation of the world into regions and nations, or economic development, allows for comparison with various others, and allows for the logic of best practice to be transposed from one region or community to another. Epidemiological data are used to measure and compare by organisations such as the Global Observatory for Physical Activity, which aims to "Reduce the global prevalence of physical inactivity among adults from 31% to 28% [and] increase indexed publications on physical activity interventions based on information and communication technology that come from low- and middle-income countries" (GOPA, 2019). Every place is a potential site for analysis.

Evangelicalism

It is surely not an exaggeration to say that physical activity is now seen in some quarters as a cure for all of society's ills. From preventing obesity, cancer, and diabetes to improving school results, giving direction to the lives of disaffected youth, and rebuilding dysfunctional communities, it is hard to think of a problem for which physical activity is not seen as a cure.

(Zanker and Gard, 2008, p. 49)

Even a superficial reading of physical activity policies reveals that physical activity is imbued with a wide range of personal and societal benefits (and increasingly wide ranging over time). Correlations between physical activity involvement and other measures such as school test scores, longevity, income, sociability and lower risks of various diseases inform much health policy. The National Health Service in the United Kingdom highlights the range of positive correlations:

It's medically proven that people who do regular physical activity have: up to a 35% lower risk of coronary heart disease and stroke, up to a 50% lower risk of type 2 diabetes, up to a 50% lower risk of colon cancer, up to a 20% lower risk of breast cancer, a 30% lower risk of early death, up to an 83% lower risk of osteoarthritis, up to a 68% lower risk of hip fracture, a 30% lower risk of falls (among older adults), up to a 30% lower risk of depression, up to a 30% lower risk of dementia.

(NHS, 2018)

While these are clearly positive benefits, the idea of physical activity has become associated with magic in popular scholarly parlance. In a 2016 editorial in the journal *Cardiology*, Lewis and Hennekens stated that "In the industrialised world today, the totality of evidence indicates that regular physical activity may have the closest resemblance to a magic bullet" (p. 360). Similarly, writing in the journal *Heart*, Coenen (2018) wrote that "Physical activity is widely considered a magic bullet for the prevention of several non-communicable (e.g., cardiovascular) diseases." (p. 1165). Similar sentiments are echoed throughout numerous conferences devoted to physical activity.

Demonisation

Evangelicalism can stray into demonisation. While the act of sitting is important for rest (energy conservation), eating and conversation and concentration on certain tasks, it has been transformed in recent years into a lethal threat. Research findings on sedentary behaviours find their way into mass media with particularly dramatic headlines. The short-lived 'Move1Hour' physical activity campaign produced advertisements which appeared around the UK claiming that "sitting is the new enemy" (Move1Hour, 2014).

Human rights

Increasingly informing the health discourse of physical activity is rhetoric of 'human rights'. The explicit ideas of human rights did not appear in the WHO 2004 physical activity strategy (WHO, 2004), but a "human rights approach" is listed as the first guiding principle of the 2018 policy (WHO, 2018). Deploying the rhetoric of rights is powerful. It suggests some consensus regarding the issue and implies safety and security for the rights holder. However, is physical activity a human right? It is not explicitly written as such in the UN Declaration of Human Rights (United Nations, 1948). (Interestingly, *rest* appears as a human right.) Ideas connected to physical activity do feature in the Declaration, such as leisure, health, education and freedom of movement (in reference to movement within nations and across borders). However, 'physical activity' does not specifically feature. And so for now, physical activity is connected to human rights by way of its connection with more specific human rights.

A better future

While many of the characteristics sketched out above could be potentially problematic, it is assumed people involved in health promotion (even in corporations) have benevolent intent. They want people to be healthier, to live longer, to have less chronic disease, and all the co-benefits often connected with physical activity – environments more conducive to community cohesion, less crime, less pollution, and so on. This benevolence can of course, be hijacked by interests, which are often corporate and which are motivated more by consumption and financial profit than health promotion.

Conclusion

Taking these discourses into account, physical activity has emerged as a legitimate policy discourse (though perhaps not yet a discipline). A range of justifications are used to legitimise intervention. By correlating insufficient physical inactivity with all manner of economic, health, environmental and interpersonal outcomes, there are a number of flow-on effects which themselves aid in sustaining and growing the physical activity political discourse:

- New reasons for promoting physical activity can be identified and promoted.
- New experts can be ratified and endorsed.
- New technology can be produced and marketed to ensure that individuals are made cognisant of their daily physical activity levels and made loyal to brands which help track them.
- States and companies can provide guidelines and encouragement to the inactive populace.
- Transnational organisations can be legitimated, such as the International Council for Sport Science and Physical Education (ICSSPE), the International Society for Physical Activity and Health (ISPAH), and the American College of Sports Medicine (ACSM).
- Academic departments and positions can be established, most usually in the area of 'physical activity and health' (as distinct from physical education), bringing physical activity as a trans-disciplinary pursuit into universities.

And so this discourse produces new experts, new expectations, authoritative organisations and social ordering. To capture the breadth of domains and knowledges which focus on physical activity, I propose the term *exerceology*. It encapsulates the totality of study, surveillance and promotion of physical activity for a wide variety of outcomes. *Exerceology* encompasses the swirling mass of concern for physical activity, from the governmental concerns of states to decrease NCD rates, to the logics and interest frames embraced by community groups and corporations alike.

References

All Party Commission on Physical Activity [APCPA] (2014). *Tackling Physical Inactivity: A Co-ordinated Approach.* England, UK: APCPA.

Blair, S.N. (2009). Physical inactivity: The biggest public health problem of the 21st century. *British Journal of Sports Medicine*, *43*, 1–2.

Christen, M. and Schmidt, S. (2012). A formal framework for conceptions of sustainability: A theoretical contribution to the discourse in sustainable development. *Sustainable Development*, *20*, 400–410.

Coenen, P. (2018). Preventing disease by integrating physical activity in clinical practice: What works for whom? *Heart*, *104*, 1140–1141.

Dallaire, C., Lemyre, L., Krewski, D. and Gibbs, L.B. (2012). The gap between knowing and doing: How Canadians understand physical activity as a health risk management strategy. *Sociology of Sport Journal*, *29*(3), 325–347.

Das, P. and Horton, R. (2016). Physical activity: Time to take it seriously and regularly. *The Lancet*, 388, 1254–1255.

Ding, D., Lawson, K.D., Kolbe-Alexander, T.L., Finkelstein, E.A., Katzmarzyk, P.T., van Mechelen, W. and Pratt, M. (2016). The economic burden of physical inactivity: A global analysis of major non-communicable diseases. *The Lancet, 388*(10051), 1311–1324.

DOH (2009). *Change4Life Principles and Guidelines for Promotion.* London: UK Department of Health.

Edwards, L.C., Bryant, A.S., Keegan, R.J., Morgan, K. and Jones, A.M. (2017). Definitions, foundations and associations of physical literacy: A systematic review. *Sports Medicine, 47,* 113.

Fitzpatrick, K. and Tinning, R. (eds) (2014). *Health Education: Critical Perspectives.* London: Routledge.

Foucault, M. (1970). *The Order of Things: An Archaeology of the Human Sciences.* London: Tavistock.

Foucault, M. (1972). *The Archaeology of Knowledge.* United Kingdom: Routledge.

Foucault, M. (1980). The politics of health in the eighteenth century. In C. Gordon (ed.), *Power/Knowledge: Selected Interviews and Other Writings 1972–1977* (pp. 166–182). Harlow, England: Harvester Press.

Foucault, M. (1994). Governmentality. In J. Faubion (ed.), *Michel Foucault: Power, Essential Works of Foucault 1954–1984*, Vol. 3 (pp. 201–222). London: Penguin.

Gard, M., and Vander Schee, C. (2014). Schools, the state and public health: Some historical and contemporary insights. In K. Fitzpatrick and R. Tinning (eds), *Health Education: Critical Perspectives* (pp. 61–74). Abingdon, Oxon, United Kingdom: Routledge.

Gard, M. and Wright, J. (2005). *The Obesity Epidemic: Science, Morality and Ideology.* Great Britain: Routledge.

GOPA (2019). Goals. Retrieved from www.globalphysicalactivityobservatory.com/

Guthold, R., Stevens, G.A., Riley, L.M. and Bull, F.C. (2018). Worldwide trends in insufficient physical activity from 2001 to 2016: A pooled analysis of 358 population-based surveys with 1·9 million participants. *Lancet Global Health.*

Hall, S. (1997). The work of representation. In S. Hall (ed.), *Representation: Cultural Representations and Signifying Practices* (pp. 13–74). Thousand Oaks, CA: Sage.

Hallal, P.C., Bauman, A.E., Heath, G.W., Kohl, H.W., Lee, I. and Pratt, M. (2012). Physical activity: More of the same is not enough. *The Lancet, 380*(9838), 190–191.

Jung, H., Pope, S. and Kirk, D. (2016). Policy for physical education and school sport in England, 2003–2010: Vested interests and dominant discourses. *Physical Education and Sport Pedagogy, 21*(5), 501–516.

Kohl, H.W., Craig, C.L., Lambert, E.V., Inoue, S., Alkandari, J.R., Leetongin, G. and Kahlmeier, S., for the Lancet Physical Activity Series Working Group (2012). The pandemic of physical inactivity: Global action for public health. *The Lancet, 380*(9838), 294–305.

Lee, I.-M., Shiroma, E.J., Lobelo, F., Puska, P., Blair, S.N. and Katzmarzyk, P.T., for the Lancet Physical Activity Series Working Group (2012). Effect of physical inactivity on major noncommunicable diseases worldwide: An analysis of burden of disease and life expectancy. *The Lancet, 380*(9838), 219–229.

Lewis, S.F. and Hennekens, C.H. (2016). Regular physical activity: A 'magic bullet' for the pandemics of obesity and cardiovascular disease. *Cardiology, 134*(3), 360–363.

Lupton, D. (2012). M-health and health promotion: The digital cyborg and surveillance society. *Social Theory and Health, 10*(3), 229–244.

Markula, P. and Pringle, R. (2006). *Foucault, Sport and Exercise: Power, Knowledge and Transforming the Self.* New York: Routledge.

May, T. (2018). *Letter to the Nation*, 24 November. 10 Downing St.

Move1Hour (2014). Move1Hour physical activity campaign. Retrieved from https://twitter.com/move1hour

NHS (2018). Benefits of exercise. Retrieved from www.nhs.uk/live-well/exercise/exercise-health-benefits/

O'Connor, A. (2015, 1 December). Research group funded by Coca-Cola to disband. *New York Times*. Retrieved from https://well.blogs.nytimes.com/2015/12/01/research-group-funded-by-coca-cola-to-disband/

Petersen, A.R. and Lupton, D. (1996). *The New Public Health: Discourses, Knowledges, Strategies.* Allen and Unwin: Australia.

Pronger, B. (2002). *Body Fascism: Salvation in the Technology of Physical Fitness.* Toronto: University of Toronto Press.

Public Health England (2014). *Everybody Active, Every Day: An Evidence-based Approach to Physical Activity.* London: Public Health England.

Scheurich, J. (1994). Policy archaeology: A new policy studies methodology. *Journal of Education Policy, 9*(4), 297–316.

Scheurich, J. (1997). *Research Method in the Postmodern.* London: Falmer Press.

Shoemaker, P.J., Tankard Jr, J.W. and Lasorsa, D.L. (2003). *How to Build Social Science Theories.* Thousand Oaks, CA: Sage Publications.

Smith Maguire, J. (2002). Michel Foucault: Sport, power and governmentality. In J. Maguire and K. Young (eds), *Theory, Sport and Society* (pp. 295–314). Amsterdam, Boston: JAI.

Tinning, R. (2010). *Pedagogy and Human Movement: Theory, Practice, Research.* London: Routledge.

United Nations (1948). Universal Declaration of Human Rights. Retrieved from www.un.org/en/universal-declaration-human-rights/

WHO (2004). *Global Strategy on Diet, Physical Activity and Health.* Geneva: World Health Organisation.

WHO (2018). *Global Action Plan on Physical Activity 2018–2030: More Active People for a Healthier World.* Geneva: World Health Organisation.

Zanker, C. and Gard, M. (2008). Fatness, fitness, and the moral universe of sport and physical activity. *Sociology of Sport Journal, 25*(1), 48–65.

4 Physical activity and the politics of knowledge

Introduction[1]

In July 2012, *The Lancet* announced a pandemic of physical inactivity and a global call to action to effect change. The worldwide pandemic is said to be claiming millions of lives every year. Asserting that physical inactivity is pandemic is an important moment. Given the purported scale and significance of physical inactivity around the world, this chapter examines how the pandemic is rhetorically constructed and how various solutions are proposed. A governmentality lens is used to examine the continuity, coherence and appropriateness of ideas about physical activity. The analysis demonstrates that within *The Lancet*, there is disunity about what is known about physical activity, problematic claims of 'abnormality' and contradictions in the proposed deployment of a systems approach to solve the problem. The chapter concludes by suggesting that, as knowledge produced about physical activity grows, scholars need to beware of nostalgic conceptions of physical activity, account for the immense diversity of lived experiences which do not abide by idealistic recommendations, and consider more rigorously contentious claims about physical activity programme effects.

The promotion of health is inherently political, and it is well established that the causes of and solutions to all social problems are contested through rhetoric, discourse and narrative (Petersen and Lupton, 1996; Stone, 2002). Roe (1994) describes the importance of "metanarratives" in constructing a hegemonic approach to a specific policy issue. A metanarrative is a dominant story that is developed over time by one or more parties involved in the social problem. These stories are used to establish and stabilize the assumptions for policy making in response to the issue's uncertainty, complexity or polarization (Roe, 1994).

One recent metanarrative is the *global physical inactivity pandemic*, an important contribution to which is the *Lancet Physical Activity Series*

(Lancet, 2012). This both defines and actively constructs how 'we' (the scientific and academic communities at least and the human population at most) should think about physical activity. Understanding more about the production dynamics of physical activity knowledge is important for various reasons. How any pandemic is framed will have important consequences for proposed health outcomes and the distribution of various resources. Any such problem requires that action is taken, whether this is in the form of government funding to address the problem, new laws to decrease the prevalence of the problem, or the modification of a population's behaviour to minimise the problem (Parsons, 1995). As a lobbying tool, the pandemic is potentially very powerful, since a significant amount of resources might be directed towards measuring, scrutinising and encouraging people to behave in particular ways and for particular reasons. The ideas espoused might also govern how a range of organisations use physical activity, and influence how agents and causes are (re)framed. Further, ideas about physical activity can impact on how individuals think about the activities in which they partake and also about their own and others' bodies.

This analysis builds on the growing attention given to the various narratives and discourses through which physical activity policies and programmes are used to nudge (Vallgårda, 2011), police (Piggin *et al.*, 2007), empower (Bercovitz, 1998), inspire (Evans, 2013), exhort (Garvin and Eyles, 1997), intervene (Mansfield and Rich, 2013) and educate (Gard and Wright, 2001). It is also situated at a specific moment with regard to the obesity epidemic. Gard (2011) contends that the obesity epidemic is essentially over: "by 2010 a new phase in the obesity epidemic had been reached, marking the end of a period of consciousness raising or hyperbole … and a transitioning to something else" (p. 4). That "something else", in this case, is the physical inactivity pandemic. This new problem shifts the focus from what we are, to how we act.

Some focus has already been directed towards the ways in which ideas about public health pandemics are produced and framed (Abeysinghe and White, 2010, 2011). In research on a recent flu pandemic policy, Holmes (2010) concluded that "despite a history of critical research on constructions of disease, social sciences literature on pandemics is primarily practical" (p. iii). Holmes' research concluded that a variety of discursive elements, including active language and statistics, recalling the past as key to the future, reference to expert knowledge, and conferring moral responsibility on the public to feel at risk, constructed a pandemic flu as inevitable, significant and manageable. Regarding the framing of health debates, recent research has focused on contests between public health organisations and corporations, for example in relation to obesity (Kim and Willis,

2007; Kwan, 2009; Jenkin *et al.*, 2011). Some research exists regarding the messages of physical activity policies. In the Australian policy context Fullagar (2002) examined health promotion campaigns with regard to the rationalities and ethics through which individuals are encouraged to govern their own healthy lifestyle practices in the name of freedom. In particular she examined the ways in which individuals may come to govern their own subjectivity through 'healthy' lifestyles and leisure practices. This current analysis builds on Fullagar's work in two ways. First, the chapter investigates ideas which inform physical activity promotion at a global level. Second, the increasingly diverse interest groups beyond state governments which seek to change the behaviour of populations are incorporated. The lobbying potential of physical activity scholars is considered explicitly.

In order to understand more about the physical activity narratives involved and the rhetoric that sustains them, this analysis focuses on a specific case study which has produced a declaration of a global physical inactivity pandemic. In particular, the focus is on how knowledge is created about physical activity in the influential medical journal, *The Lancet*. Various question inform the analysis. What ideas about physical activity are foregrounded? Are these ideas coherent? Are these ideas always appropriate? The way in which facts are disseminated is also important to consider. Petersen and Lupton (1996) note that "like other scientific facts, epidemiological facts gain their credence from being published in scholarly journals, in which process the historical and sociocultural dimensions of their construction ... are effectively hidden" (p. 33). In the case of *The Lancet Series* on physical activity, the journal's reputation as a renowned health publication bestows a sense of legitimacy upon the claims made. It is these hidden and possibly unaccounted for dynamics of construction that are focused upon. It is not our goal to construct a perfect, coherent story about the history and meaning of physical activity. Rather, by exposing misrepresentations and contradictions by world-leading experts involved in *The Lancet*, the reader might become sceptical about grand proclamations, and second, develop a critical and ethical approach to physical activity promotion.

Given the purported multidimensional nature of the physical inactivity pandemic, the current examination merges a variety of methodological perspectives. Our theoretical framework is broadly informed by writings on governmentality (Rose, 1990; Rose and Miller, 1992; Foucault, 1994; Markula and Pringle, 2006). Foucault (1994) uses governmentality to describe the regulation of individuals' lives, which involves procedures, analyses, calculations and tactics that allow for the exercise of power through the governing of others. Rose (1990) goes on to note that it is through these interlocking apparatuses for the programming of various dimensions of life that we are "urged, incited, encouraged, exhorted and motivated to act" (p. xxii). Rose and Miller (1992) assert that these various forms of power are used by governments to ensure citizens believe in "a kind of regulated freedom" (p. 174). By understanding more about these dynamics (with particular regard to physical activity), one can begin to either support or question the impact of such espoused meanings and interventions in the lives of citizens. Propositions such as those put forward in *The Lancet* about physical activity provide a significant moment to examine "a whole complex of knowledges" (Foucault, 1994, p. 220).

A specific set of documents is analysed, and is limited to the *Lancet Physical Activity Series* published in July 2012. The Series consists of five 'comments', one 'article', and five further articles under the heading 'Series'. The selection of these articles for analysis is considered and deliberate, since it captures the moment of the announcement of the physical activity pandemic, the description of the 'landscape' in which to address the pandemic, the proposed actions that are needed, and the important actors and institutions. Ultimately, the aim of undertaking this analysis is to disrupt the taken-for-granted assumptions and 'facts' which 'govern' the ideas presented in *The Lancet* before any major policy initiatives are rolled out in order to combat physical inactivity. Not only may these result in the inefficient distribution of scarce resources, but potentially harm citizens' understandings about physical activity. To paraphrase Pringle and Pringle (2012), here the validity of the truth claims surrounding physical activity is critiqued while also drawing on the notion of 'health' as justification for rejecting some of the ideas proposed.

Context: *The Lancet* and the global physical inactivity pandemic

According to its own website, *The Lancet* journal is an authoritative voice in global medicine. With an 'impact factor' of 38.28 at the time of writing, which is among the highest of all academic journals, it is clearly influential in the medical community. In July 2012, *The Lancet* published a Series of physical activity commentaries and articles about the physical inactivity pandemic and called for a "social revolution ... towards an active physical and mental life" (Das and Horton, 2012, pp. 189–190).[2] The global significance of physical inactivity was highlighted on numerous occasions. The pandemic is said to be affecting all nations in the world (Das and Horton, 2012). According to the Series, "physical inactivity is the fourth leading cause of death worldwide" (Kohl *et al.*, 2012, p. 294) and is said to be responsible for "6–10% of all deaths from the major NCDs .... [and] more than 5.3% of the 57 million deaths that occurred worldwide in 2008" (Lee *at al.*, 2012, p. 219).

While *The Lancet Series* contains much large-scale quantitative data about the benefits of physical activity, it also includes a significant amount of rhetoric and argumentation to shape the physical inactivity pandemic. Claiming that physical inactivity is 'pandemic' is an important moment in health promotion discourse. It suggests a rhetorical and policy shift in attention away from physical inactivity being a component of the 'obesity epidemic', thereby requiring alterations in how population health is perceived and addressed by a range of stakeholders.

The call to action that culminates in *The Lancet Series* requires a wide array of organisations in every nation to change their practices, including transnational organisations such as the UN and WHO, national governments, companies, voluntary organisations, and academics and individuals. By considering the growing field of physical activity scholarship as a potent policy domain, this current analysis examines how the problem of the pandemic is rhetorically constructed and how solutions are proposed.

The attempted rewriting of the history of physical activity

Numerous statements in the Series use both recent and 'ancient' history as important reference points to justify focusing on physical activity. However, many of these claims fail to contain sufficient rigour in their production. In an article that provides much statistical evidence for a physical activity revolution, Lee *et al.* write:

> Ancient physicians – including those from China in 2600 BC and Hippocrates around 400 BC – believed in the value of physical activity for health. By the 20th century, however, a diametrically opposite view – that exercise was dangerous – *prevailed instead.*
>
> (p. 219, italics added)

This claim uses various rhetorical devices to create a powerful narrative about physical activity. It invokes the wisdom of the "Ancients" from Greece and China and suggests that their espousal of health practices had somehow been usurped and subjugated by forces not identified in the text. This is a powerful story of decline whereby "in the beginning, things were pretty good. But they got worse. In fact, they are nearly intolerable. Something must be done" (Stone, 2002, p. 138). However, this narrative is both inaccurate and is itself also used by other authors in the Series to propagate further misrepresentations.

First, it is unreasonable to use the twentieth century as the time during which scepticism about exercise prevailed. Further, it is inaccurate to claim that an opposing view "prevailed *instead*". Tracing the literature that Lee *et al.* use to support their own claim illuminates this. The evidence offered for the "prevailing" view that "exercise was dangerous" originated from a *British Medical Journal* article by Rook (1954) which reported on an investigation into "the longevity of Cambridge sportsmen". The article by Rook claimed that "*Many observers, both in ancient and in more modern times*, have pointed out the alleged dangers of such activities" (p. 774, italics added). In turn, Rook cites Hartley and Llewellyn (1939) who wrote that concerns have existed about strenuous exercise since "the earliest times" (p. 657). These historical debates, both ancient and recent, about the concerns about exercise are omitted by Lee *et al.* in favour of a more dramatic, though inaccurate, narrative.

The transformation of the narrative continues, when Wen and Wu (2012) use the claims by Lee *et al.* as a reference in the assertion that "Socially, being inactive is perceived as normal, and in fact doctors order patients to remain on bed rest far more often than they encourage exercise" (p. 192). This is inaccurate in two respects. First, Lee *et al.* do not claim that "being inactive is perceived as normal". Second, Lee *et al. actually* write that "During the early 20th century, complete bed rest was prescribed for patients with acute myocardial infarction" (p. 219) which is totally incongruent with Wen and Wu's assertion. It is important that the narrative regarding physical activity promotion does not include dramatic statements such as "in fact doctors order patients to remain on bed rest far more often than they encourage exercise" without supporting evidence. The problematic climax to this series of inaccuracies is the claim by Wen and Wu (2012) that "This passive attitude towards inactivity, where exercise is viewed as a personal choice, is anachronistic, and is reminiscent of the battles still being fought over smoking" (p. 192). This view is derived from a series of misrepresentations by various authors within *The Lancet*, and therefore should be treated with scepticism. These narratives are powerful to the extent that they attempt to justify the research that follows. The simplifications and misrepresentations suggest a need for a more critical approach by physical activity scholars to understanding what societies *do* think about physical activity. These grand proclamations require more rigorous consideration by the various researchers in the first instance and more scrutiny by editors and reviewers of *The Lancet* in the second.

The rhetorical technique of nostalgically referencing a bygone age is also apparent in another aspect of *The Lancet*. The cover page of *The Lancet Series* is adorned with an image (which is repeated on the first page) of a painting of what appears to be children playing. Indeed the painting is called *Children's Games* (*Kinderspiele*) from 1560, by Pieter Bruegel. The image portrays a town square full of young people playing both outside and in the surrounding buildings. The intention of including the image (twice) is to imply that populations have indeed neglected or forgotten the goodness of games.

A cursory analysis of *Children's Games*, however, reveals various activities which would surely be deemed detrimental to physical or mental health today. They include a child poking and stirring what appears to be excrement with a stick, someone urinating only a few metres from where others are playing, a group of children kicking the legs of others, another group seemingly manhandling an uncooperative person, and a child being bullied by having their hair pulled by a group of others.[3] It is unlikely this image would have been purposefully selected had this range of health-diminishing activities been recognised. The interpretation of these images here is not an argument against the wide variety of benefits that come from different types of physical activity. Instead, by drawing attention to the various, often contradictory ideas about what 'physical activity' involves it becomes clear that both hundreds of years ago, and currently, the realm of physical activity involves more than 'brisk walking'.

Also on the first page is a quote from the 'Ancient' Plato which reads "Lack of activity destroys the good condition of every human being while movement and methodical physical exercise save it and preserve it" (Das and Horton, 2012). Both the quote and a general view of the painting promote a naïvely nostalgic view of what life used to be like and advocate a return to particular traditional ideas and practices of yesteryear. It is interesting to note that the origins of nostalgia are to be found in medicine itself. As Boym points out,

> It would not occur to us to demand a prescription for nostalgia. Yet in the seventeenth century nostalgia was considered to be a curable disease, akin to a severe common cold. Swiss doctors believed that opium, leeches, and a journey to the Swiss Alps would take care of nostalgic symptoms.
>
> (2007, p. 7)

While such remedies might indeed be problematic, Boym's (2007, pp. 9–10) claim resonates; "The danger of nostalgia is that it tends to confuse the actual home with the imaginary one", in this case the past, in which premature death was a fact of life, and the imagined past in which children were physically active and, as a result, healthy.

In many cases generalisations about yesteryear and 'the Ancients' are relied upon to contextualise the issue under discussion. However, such grand summations simplify the debated and contested history of thought about physical activity. Of course, these arguments are not the main focus of *The Lancet* articles. Historical anecdotes are mostly offered as introductions to the research and policy suggestions that follow. However, this 'scene setting' is important when considering the range of claims that are made about what is, or is not appropriate physical activity. Despite these contrary statements mentioned above, as rhetorical devices, all of the claims contribute to a narrative that something must be done. In the course of doing so, the claims rule in and rule out certain types of action and certain types of knowledges which can be used to regulate the behaviour of a population. This is explored in the next section.

Abnormal, design and failure: the politics of regulating populations

In both subtle and explicit ways, particular types of physical activity are promoted and marginalised in *The Lancet*. Foucault referred to these as dividing practices; "the judges of normality are present everywhere. We're in the society of the teacher-judge, the doctor-judge.... It is on them that the universal reign of the normative is based..." (Foucault, 1979, p. 304). Here are considerations of which ideas are promoted as acceptable (or "normal") in the Series.

In the final call to action, Kohl *et al.* claim that "The freedom and opportunity for individuals to participate in physical activity should be viewed as a basic human right" (p. 300). "Freedom" is a wholly worthwhile principle, and in one significant way, it is addressed in a Series article by Rimmer and Marques entitled 'Physical activity for people with disabilities' (p. 193). Rimmer and Marques propose that more is done to promote physical activity for the more than one billion people worldwide who have disabilities. However, while ideas about "freedom" and "rights" do feature, there are also other ideas which work against these ideas. For example, there are instances where "normality" is referred to in a way which deviates from other, more inclusive discourse. Attention is focused in particular on Wen and Wu's suggestion that

> In addition to doctors' traditional advocacy of the health benefits of exercise, stressing that the harms of inactivity could strengthen our battle against inactivity. *We need to view the inactive population as abnormal* and consider them at high risk of disease.
>
> (p. 193, italics added)[4]

Describing people as "abnormal" when considering physical activity promotion is wholly inappropriate. This idea is particularly worrying. The plethora of literature which exists around problematic aspects of the obesity epidemic alone should alert us to the possibility of stigma associated with being labelled as inactive (see Gard and Wright, 2005; Puhl, 2011; Puhl and King, 2013). In their *Lancet* text, Wen and Wu also state:

> To individuals, *the failure* to spend 15–30 min a day in brisk walking increases the risk of cancer, heart disease, stroke, and diabetes by 20–30%, and shortens lifespan by 3–5 years.
>
> (p. 192, italics added)

In a similarly normative manner, Das and Horton state that the Series is concerned with

> using the body that we have in the way it was designed, which is to walk often, run sometimes, and move in ways where we physically exert ourselves regularly whether that is at work, at home, in transport to and from places, or during leisure time in our daily lives.
>
> (p. 189)

These quotes are concerning for two reasons. First, using "15–30 min a day in brisk walking" is overly normative, and does not reflect the range of disabilities which people around the world face. Any promotion of physical activity should extend to people who, for a wide variety of reasons, can neither walk nor run. Second, the idea that individuals "fail" at this task is in total opposition to a systems approach advocated by many of the authors in the Series who focus more on structural factors.[5] In light of the significant attention given to promoting surveillance within the Series, reflection is needed with regard to people who, no matter how they were "designed", do not obey these normative descriptions and prescriptions. There is surely space for physical activity scholars to produce more inclusive definitions of what physical activity can be. These definitions should take into account ideas about diversity of movement as well as the diverse meanings attached to physical activity. Scholars in physical education and pedagogy have demonstrated time and again that they are willing to be self-critical and to examine new ways in which physical activity among young people can be increased and improved (see Quennerstedt, 2008). As Stidder (2013) notes, "critical self-reflection and pedagogy through the use of reflexivity in physical education can contextualise and illustrate various topics of educational debate as well as inform research and provide the impetus for innovation and change" (p. 19). There is little evidence to date of such self-analysis among the overwhelming majority of physical activity scholars who might consider the evidence base for some of their espoused truths.

Foucault writes that there are powerful effects of claims about normality: "each individual, wherever he [*sic*] may find himself, subjects to [normative ideas] his body, his gestures, his behavior, his aptitudes, his achievements" (Foucault, 1979, p. 304). While regular physical activity might indeed contribute to healthy, able bodies, physical activity scholars would benefit from integrating the diversity of human life more fully into their proclamations. There is space in the domain of physical activity policy "for further consideration with respect to how to talk about the fit body" (Neville, 2013, p. 490).

Normality, of course, is imbued with judgement and evaluation. And this is where surveillance becomes justifiable and yet potentially invasive. Regarding surveillance, a claim is made in *The Lancet* by Kohl *et al.* that a "*complete understanding* of all stakeholders, their interactions, and how their interactions make up the whole is crucial to understanding of the systems that impede progress on physical activity" (p. 302, italics added). While the goal of attaining "complete understanding" is ultimately futile, it is disturbing that this would be a goal at all. And so more questions arise. What does "complete" mean in the physical activity domain? What knowledge about individuals is "fair game" for physical activity researchers pursuing this goal? What surveillance techniques might be utilised to attain this "complete understanding"? Where do individual rights fit in with such a plan? These questions must be given attention by physical activity scholars, particularly since ideas about surveillance also feature prominently in the Series.

Olympic Legacy claims: denial, lamentation or praiseworthy?

While many organisations are integrated into *The Lancet*'s call to action, there is a significant amount of attention given to the International Olympic Committee and the Olympics Games. Throughout the Series, however, it is clear that there is much contention about the value of the Olympic Games in promoting physical activity. This case of rhetoric about the Olympic Games demonstrates that even though various *Lancet* authors promote a systems approach, the complexity of any issue can become so great as to stifle any positive action. Hallal *et al.* unequivocally claim that

> The popularity of the Olympic Games and elite sports such as professional soccer *has not been, and will not be, translated into mass participation in exercise and physical activity* that will improve the health of the world's population.
>
> (p. 190, italics added)

Refuting the claim that worldwide physical activity from the Olympic Games will occur is a powerful rhetorical device. It adds to the problem, since it alerts the reader to the possibility that some aims are not being achieved (despite the fact that no person or organisation is cited as having made the claim in the first place). This denial differs from *The Lancet* editorial for the Series, which suggests that the Olympic Games are actually *detrimental* to health. The editorial criticises the involvement of sponsors such as Coca Cola, Cadbury's and McDonald's and laments "the long-term effect of Games-associated junk food advertising on people's hearts and waistlines – definitely one Olympic legacy the world can do without" (p. 188).

This 'villain' narrative is certainly popular, although a critical ecological approach might consider two problematic aspects of this view. First, the tone of these claims about the "Olympic effect" differs significantly from that of another commentary in the Series in which Malta and Silva write about efforts in Brazil to promote physical activity using the Olympic Games. They write that "the Brazilian government launched a strategic plan to tackle NCDs in 2011" (Malta and Silva, 2012, p. 196). Part of this strategic plan is to use the 2016 Olympic Games to promote physical activity:

> Furthermore, educational measures that foster healthy habits and the practice of daily physical activity are underway as part of the legacy of two major sporting events that will be held in Brazil: the 2014 World Cup and the Olympic Games in 2016.
>
> (p. 196)

Adding to the contention about the value of the Olympic Games, in the final call to action this Brazilian strategic plan is *praised*,

> Ideally, national policies and action plans are designed not for implementation solely by governments, but rather for mobilisation of both governmental and non-governmental collaboration towards advancement of physical activity and reduction of physical inactivity. The recent Brazilian experience is one from which many such lessons can be learned. Similar action is needed worldwide.
>
> (Kohl *et al.*, p. 296)

What all of this highlights, among other things, is a failure to engage with research conducted by social scientists into legacy issues associated with the Olympic Games and other mega events. Long before the London Olympics of 2012 took place, it was being pointed out that, if large-scale changes in sports participation were to occur, these would be the consequence of interaction between numerous factors, including improved infrastructure for grass-roots activities (Coalter, 2004). Any suggestion that simply by hosting a mega event, such interaction will inevitably follow is idealistic in the extreme. Post-2012, there is little evidence that youth sport participation has increased since the Games. As Judy Murray, mother of British tennis gold-medal winner Andy, has pointed out, there is a dearth of new talent in her sport not least because several schemes to improve free-to-use public courts in deprived urban areas have failed to materialise (Parkhouse, 2013). Inspiring a generation, which was the aim of London 2012, is one thing but if there are insufficient facilities and coaches to meet demand, the inspired generation will become quickly disillusioned. In addition, figures show that "there are now fewer adults playing sport regularly than before the London 2012 Olympics" (Gibson, 2013). Indeed, as Bell (2013, p. 175) concludes, "despite the excitement and interest London 2012 generated, delivering an inspirational and successful Olympics/Paralympics was not sufficient on its own to get more people taking part in sport – as many had already predicted". None of this is to suggest that participation levels will never increase after the staging of a mega event, such as the Olympic Games. The point is, however, that apparently unbeknown to some *Lancet* authors, there has long been a significant and well-informed debate on such matters which they ignore to their detriment.[6]

The Lancet statements illuminate not only the stark contradictions that characterise the debate about the 'Olympic effect' but also reveal that some of these contradictions come from authors in the same Lancet Physical Activity Series Working Group. To extrapolate this point, the sentiments of denial and lamentation above cannot be reconciled with the advice in the climatic "call to action" article which encourages the private sector to:

> Orient marketing, advertising, and promotional messages to encourage physical activity and discourage physical inactivity and sedentary behaviours [and] collaborate with government and non-governmental organisations in the creation and promotion of opportunities to promote and engage in physical activity.
>
> (Kohl *et al.*, p. 302)

That is, the call to action specifically *encourages* private companies to promote physical activity. This case demonstrates the non-linear and multi-faceted nature of appeals to 'health'. It also illustrates the governmental forces at work, whereby there are interlocking (but not necessarily synergistic) apparatuses which contribute to lived environments. These apparatuses "form a force field through which we are urged, incited, encouraged, exhorted and motivated to act" (Rose, 1990, p. xxii). One might argue that *The Lancet Series* does promote acknowledging these multifaceted understandings through a systems approach. In their call to action, Kohl *et al.* argue that a variety of "different areas are needed to tackle the global pandemic of physical inactivity because multidisciplinary work is essential" (p. 294). However, a more concerted systems approach would acknowledge this paradox of the Olympics as at once hindering and assisting health in order to establish a more nuanced appreciation of the complexities associated with corporate sponsorship of sport events. Certainly, these paradoxes demonstrate the need for urgent review focused on existing policies and practices. By acknowledging the multiplicity of these corporate and non-governmental arrangements, a more "ecological" context can be presented.

Conclusion

While the Physical Activity Series is well-intended, there remain concerns regarding the continuity, coherence and appropriateness of various ideas that emanate from it. The idea of encouraging people to partake in more physical activity is to be applauded. However, the complexities inherent within the global pandemic metanarrative disrupt the possibility of rigorous argument. The concerns expressed here are not intended to derail momentum being generated in relation to physically active lifestyles. Instead, by giving more rigorous attention to defining and discussing the context and meanings of physical activity, fairer, more respectful and more effective promotion can result. The institutionalised, population-wide study of physical activity is relatively new, and, as Bull and Bauman note, physical inactivity might be described as the "Cinderella" of NCD risk factors, with a "poverty of policy attention and resourcing proportionate to its importance" (p. 13). There is clearly space then, for physical activity scholars to reflect on what stories are being (and should be) told about physical activity, in order to develop a more nuanced approach to engaging with it.

The Lancet Series frames the physical inactivity pandemic as complex. Claiming a social problem is complex allows for it to be conceived, explained and measured in particular ways, in this case requiring a "systems approach" (Kohl *et al.*, p. 294) or an "ecological" model (Bauman *et al.*, p. 258). According to Kohl *et al.*:

> a systems approach acknowledges the complex non-linearity of health behaviours, including the many interactions, delays in adoption,

adaptations, competing actions, and unintended consequences that can occur within a system. A systems approach acknowledges such complexities and allows for planning to counteract the unintended consequences.

(p. 300)

A systems approach would also need to account for and attempt to mitigate the complexities, competing ideas and unintended consequences inherent within its own propositions. It is apparent that various authors in *The Lancet* make bold, definitive and binary claims about physical activity and sport. These claims are of significant import given their possible influence in public health policy formulation and subsequent resource allocation. However, not only are these claims at times contradictory, but they are difficult to reconcile with a proposed systems approach which purportedly aims to consider unintended effects. Various claims acknowledge the complexity of social life (such as Kohl *et al.* suggesting even a well-designed intervention might result in a "net zero gain" due to unintended consequences). At other times, however, complexity is dismissed in favour of grand generalisations and definitions.

The ways in which the Physical Activity Series is transformed into policy and practice are yet to be seen. Given that physical activity is indeed a complex arena, physical activity researchers should be cautioned to avoid elevating any physical health justifications for engaging in physical activity above other meanings that motivate people to be active. Using walking as one example, Bairner (2012) argued the physical health benefits accrued from walking "may well be of secondary importance to the lessons that can be learned from the pedagogies of the street" (p. 373). Therefore, at the very least, physical activity promoters should not lose sight of the benefits and meanings of certain activities simply because they lack physical exertion. To reiterate Fullagar's (2002) remarks: "What is at stake here is the way that health policy discourses do or do not engage with other logics and modes of embodiment when promoting active leisure as something more than a risk-reducing physical activity" (p. 73). More consideration of the implications of adopting a systems approach is needed before advancing the call to action further. There is space to consider Mansfield and Rich's (2013) suggestion of institutional "border crossings" by physical activity scholars so that "counter perspectives and critical voices offering alternative health paradigms" (p. 356) will not be systematically marginalised or silenced.

This analysis provides an opportunity to acknowledge the dangers of what is at times a totalising response, particularly regarding surveillance. What is required is a weighing up of competing values (such as 'complete understanding' versus privacy) and competing stories (such as the various histories of health). Although *The Lancet* is undoubtedly a world leading medical journal, it is not the only, or even the dominant, producer of truth about physical activity. Academic journals are situated within a wider milieu of diverse truth claims, institutions, cultures and histories. There is a vast array of issues, a myriad of organisations and a complex nexus of research, policies, treatments and behaviours involved in managing population health around the world. The Series' ideas will only be influential to the extent populations can be mobilised by a willing 'activity-force'. The Series' call to action is not rejected here. Rather, it should be reformed.

Notes

1 This chapter is based on research by Joe Piggin and Alan Bairner (2016) published in *Sport, Education and Society*.
2 Eight years earlier in 2004, Manson *et al.* also announced escalating global pandemics of sedentary lifestyles and inactivity and also wrote a "call to action" for clinicians (Manson *et al.*, 2004).
3 Lupton (1995) notes that "from medieval times well into the closing years of the Victorian era, European towns and cities were characterised by filthy streets littered with human and animal excrement and rotting garbage" (p. 26).
4 The term 'normal' also appears in other places as common sense. Wen and Wu claim that "being inactive is perceived as *normal*" (p. 192, italics added). Lee *et al.* also imagine "if all obese people in the USA were to attain *normal* weight" (p. 228, italics added).
5 The idea of "failure" features in a profile interview in another Series in *The Lancet*, where one author makes a specific claim about physical education; "The truth is that physical educators have failed … Physical education itself hasn't delivered physical activity benefits to children in schools" (Khan, in Holmes, 2012, p. 20). This type of accusation in a world-leading medical journal that physical educators have failed has been responded to by physical education scholars as being the pursuit of not only illusory but also dangerous ideals (see Evans *et al.*, 2004).
6 Also, a systems approach would cast a critical eye over the alleged altruism of the International Olympic Committee, an organisation which has been subject to a range of critiques focused on corruption which would surely undermine its capacity to promote physical activity around the world (Lenskyj, 2008; Jennings, 2011).

References

Abeysinghe, S. and White, K. (2010). Framing disease: The avian influenza pandemic in Australia. *Health Sociology Review*, *19*, 369–381.
Abeysinghe, S. and White, K. (2011). The avian influenza pandemic: Discourses of risk, contagion and preparation in Australia. *Health, Risk & Society*, *13*(4), 311–326.

Bairner, A. (2012). Urban walking and the pedagogies of the street. *Sport, Education and Society*, *16*(3), 371–384.

Bauman, A.E., Reis, R.S., Sallis, J.F., Wells, J.C., Loos, R.J.F. and Martin, B.W., for the Lancet Physical Activity Series Working Group (2012). Correlates of physical activity: Why are some people physically active and others not? *The Lancet*, *380*(9838), 258–271.

Bell, B. (2013). From podium to park. In Mark Perryman (ed.), *London 2012. How Was It For Us?* (pp. 164–176). London: Lawrence and Wishart.

Bercovitz, K. (1998). Canada's Active Living policy: A critical analysis. *Health Promotion International*, *13*(4), 319–328.

Boym, S. (2007). Nostalgia and its discontents. *The Hedgehog Review*, Summer, 7–18.

Bruegel, P. (1560). *Kinderspiele (Children's Games)*, (oil on panel). Kunsthistorisches Museum, Vienna, Austria/The Bridgeman Art Library.

Bull, F.C. and Bauman, A.E. (2011). Physical inactivity: The 'Cinderella' risk factor for noncommunicable disease prevention. *Journal of Health Communication: International Perspectives*, *16*(sup2), 13–26.

Coalter, F. (2004). Stuck in the blocks? A sustainable sporting legacy. In A. Vigor, M. Mean and C. Tims (eds), *After the Goldrush: A Sustainable Olympics for London* (pp. 93–108). London: ippr and Demos.

Das, P. and Horton, R. (2016). Physical activity: Time to take it seriously and regularly. *The Lancet*, *388*, 1254–1255.

Evans, J. (2013). Physical Education as porn! *Physical Education and Sport Pedagogy*, *18*(1), 75–89.

Evans, J., Rich, E. and Davies, B. (2004). The emperor's new clothes: fat, thin, and overweight. The social fabrication of risk and ill health. *Journal of Teaching in Physical Education*, *23*, 372–391.

Foucault, M. (1979). *Discipline and Punish: The Birth of the Prison*. Harmondsworth: Penguin Books.

Foucault, M. (1994). Governmentality. In J. Faubion (ed.), *Michel Foucault: Power, Essential Works of Foucault 1954–1984*, Vol. 3 (pp. 201–222). London: Penguin.

Fullagar, S. (2002), Governing the healthy body: Discourses of leisure and lifestyle within Australian health policy. *Health*, *6*(1), 69–84.

Gard, M. (2011). *The End of the Obesity Epidemic*. London, Routledge.

Gard, M. and Wright, J. (2001). Managing uncertainty: Obesity discourses and physical education in a risk society. *Studies in Philosophy and Education*, *20*, 535–549.

Gard, M. and Wright, J. (eds) (2005). *The Obesity Epidemic: Science and Ideology*. London: Routledge.

Garvin, T. and Eyles, J. (1997). The sun safety metanarrative: Translating science into public health discourse. *Policy Sciences*, *30*, 47–70.

Gibson, O. (2013). Fewer adults playing sport since London Olympics. *Guardian*, 14 June. Retrieved from http://aggregga.com/kennethp80/post/632080/fewer-adults-playing-sport-since-london-olympics.

Hallal, P.C., Bauman, A.E., Heath, G.W., Kohl, H.W., Lee, I. and Pratt, M. (2012). Physical activity: More of the same is not enough. *The Lancet, 380*(9838), 190–191.

Hartley, P.H.-S. and Llewellyn, G.F. (1939). An investigation into the longevity of Cambridge sportsmen. *British Medical Journal, 1,* 657.

Holmes, B. (2010). *Constructing the Coming Plague: A Discourse Analysis of the British Columbia Pandemic Influenza Preparedness Plan*. Doctoral Thesis, Simon Fraser University. Retrieved from http://summit.sfu.ca/item/11398

Holmes, D. (2012). Profile: Karim Khan: good sport. *The Lancet, 380*(9836), 20.

Jenkin, G., Signal, L. and Thomson, G. (2011). Framing obesity: The framing contest between industry and public health at the New Zealand inquiry into obesity. *Obesity Reviews, 12,* 1022–1030.

Jennings, A. (2011). Investigating corruption in corporate sport: The IOC and FIFA. *International Review for the Sociology of Sport,* 46(4), 387–398.

Kim, S. and Willis, L. (2007). Talking about obesity: News framing of who is responsible for causing and fixing the problem. *Journal of Health Communication, 12,* 359–376.

Kohl, H.W., Craig, C.L., Lambert, E.V., Inoue, S., Alkandari, J.R., Leetongin, G. and Kahlmeier, S., for the Lancet Physical Activity Series Working Group (2012). The pandemic of physical inactivity: Global action for public health. *The Lancet, 380*(9838), 294–305.

Kwan, S. (2009). Framing the fat body: Contested meanings between government, activists, and industry. *Social Inquiry, 79,* 25–50.

The Lancet (2012). Chariots of Fries. *The Lancet, 380*(9838), 188.

Lee, I.M., Shiroma, E.J., Lobelo, F., Puska, P., Blair, S.N. and Katzmarzyk, P.T., for the Lancet Physical Activity Series Working Group (2012). Effect of physical inactivity on major non-communicable diseases worldwide: An analysis of burden of disease and life expectancy. *The Lancet, 380*(9838), 219–229.

Lenskyj, H.J. (2008). *Olympic Industry Resistance: Challenging Olympic Power and Propaganda*. New York: State University of New York Press.

Lupton, D. (1995). *The Imperative of Health Public Health and the Regulated Body*. Australia: Sage Publication Ltd.

Malta, D.C. and Silva, J.B. (2012). Policies to promote physical activity in Brazil. *The Lancet, 380*(9838), 195–196.

Mansfield, L. and Rich, E. (2013). Public health pedagogy, border crossings and physical activity at every size. *Critical Public Health, 23,* 356–370.

Manson, J.E., Skerrett, P.J., Greenland, P. and VanItallie, T.B. (2004). The escalating pandemics of obesity and sedentary lifestyle: A call to action for clinicians. *Archives of Internal Medicine, 164*(3), 249–258.

Markula, P. and Pringle, R. (2006). *Foucault, Sport and Exercise: Power, Knowledge and Transforming the Self.* New York: Routledge.

Neville, R.D. (2013). Considering a complemental model of health and fitness. *Sociology of Health & Illness, 35*(3), 479–492.

Parkhouse, S. (2013). Judy Murray: Lack of free courts is keeping tennis elitist. *The Observer,* 23 June. Retrieved from www.guardian.co.uk/sport/2013/jun/23/judy-murray-elitist-tennis

Parsons, W. (1995). *Public Policy.* Aldershot: Edward Elgar.

Petersen, A.R. and Lupton, D. (1996). *The New Public Health: Discourses, Knowledges, Strategies.* Allen and Unwin: Australia.

Piggin, J. and Bairner, A. (2014). The global physical inactivity pandemic: An analysis of knowledge production. *Sport, Education and Society, 21*(2), 131–147.

Piggin, J., Jackson, S. and Lewis, M. (2007). Classify, divide and conquer: Shaping physical activity discourse through national public policy. *New Zealand Sociology, 22*(2), 274–293.

Pringle, R. and Pringle, D. (2012). Competing obesity discourses and critical challenges for health and physical educators. *Sport, Education and Society, 17*(2), 143–161.

Puhl, R.M. (2011). Weight stigmatization toward youth: A significant problem in need of societal solutions. *Childhood Obesity, 7*(5), 359–363.

Puhl, R.M. and King, K.M. (2013). Weight discrimination and bullying. *Best Practice & Research Clinical Endocrinology & Metabolism.* Retrieved from http://dx.doi.org/10.1016/j.beem.2012.12.002

Quennerstedt, M. (2008). Exploring the relation between physical activity and health: A salutogenic approach to physical education. *Sport, Education and Society, 13*(3), 267–283.

Rimmer, J.H. and Marques, A.C. (2012). Physical activity for people with disabilities. *The Lancet, 380*(9838), 193–195.

Roe, E. (1994). *Narrative Policy Analysis: Theory and Practice.* Durham: Duke University Press.

Rook, A. (1954). An investigation into the longevity of Cambridge sportsmen. *British Medical Journal, 1,* 773–777.

Rose, N. (1990). *Governing the Soul: The Shaping of the Private Self.* London: Routledge.

Rose, N. and Miller, P. (1992). Political power beyond the state: Problematics of government. *British Journal of Sociology, 43*(2), 173–205.

Stone, D. (2002). *Policy Paradox: The Art of Political Decision Making.* New York: W.W. Norton.

Stidder, G. (2013). The value of reflexivity for inclusive practice in physical education. In G. Stidder and S. Hayes (eds), *Equity and Inclusion in Physical Education and Sport.* Second Edition (pp. 17–33). London: Routledge.

Vallgårda, S. (2011). Nudge: A new and better way to improve health? *Health Policy, 104,* 200–203.

Wen, C.P. and Wu, X. (2012). Stressing harms of physical inactivity to promote exercise. *The Lancet, 380*(9838), 192–193.

5 Physical activity and the politics of societal change

How should we be physically active? How should our cities be organised? Which activities should be prescribed and encouraged? This chapter explores how archetypal thinking can influence physical activity policies. Processes of homogenisation should not be understated. Physical activity promoters must tread carefully when elevating certain structures as ideal and certain activities as preferred or desired. Caution is warranted not only to avoid accusations of practices being imposed on a community and potential for marginalising traditional customs and practices within a local context, but also because some policy changes might be simply unachievable, and therefore inappropriate. This chapter examines the assumptions of various physical activity promoters to understand more about the dynamics of physical activity policy production. First, is an examination of how an apparently successful country's template (Finland) was attempted to be transposed onto another inactive country (the United Kingdom). Second, a recent case study of the World Health Organisation's physical activity strategy is used to explore some of the values that inform international advocacy for physical activity promotion.

Discussion about physical inactivity has escalated in recent years such that it is now positioned as a serious health problem, contributing to millions of deaths worldwide every year (Kohl *et al.*, 2012). Not only has physical inactivity been called as dangerous as smoking, but there are also a growing number of positive social, economic and health outcomes that come from being regularly physically active (Bailey *et al.*, 2013).The problem is framed as "complex", with a wide array of organisations, justifications, measurement techniques, and targeted groups being identified as important in contributing to the solution (Kohl *et al.*, 2012). Organisations ranging from governments to companies, schools, sport clubs and transport organisations means that physical inactivity cannot be situated in one place. Because of the array of places and spaces in which people might be inactive, physical inactivity is framed as a problem that affects 'everyone', and government departments around the world are increasingly formulating policy responses as a result of its significance.

Case study 1: the UK and Finland

The United Kingdom, a relatively liberal society, has seen an intensification of attention about physical activity. With physical inactivity gaining prominence in recent years as an influential public health risk factor, both state funded organisations such as the Department of Health, and non-state actors such as charities and companies have increasingly lobbied for and promoted physical activity. In 2014 specifically, a range of physical activity 'calls to action' have been published by different organisations. Four such documents were published by UKActive, the UK Government, an 'unofficial' government taskforce called the All Party Commission on Physical Activity, and Public Health England. These documents frame the problem, and to varying degrees, promote solutions. All the documents identify causes, statistics, organisations which are important in order to accomplish the goals of the documents, as denoted by their titles: 'turning the tide of (or tackling) inactivity, moving more and (therefore) living more, and getting everybody active, every day' (*Turning the Tide of Inactivity* (UKActive, 2014); *Tackling Physical Inactivity* (APCPA, 2014); *Moving More, Living More* (UK Government, 2014); and *Everybody Active, Every Day* (Public Health England, 2014)).

Given the purported societal and individual costs and benefits of inactivity, critiquing the formation of solutions will enable policy makers and scholars to better understand the dynamics involved in addressing this multifaceted, multisectoral policy issue. This analysis used comparative policy analysis to trace commonalities, distinctions, and principles for achieving proposed change in the United Kingdom (Engeli and Allison, 2014; Vallgårda, 2007, 2011). In particular it was conducted at a particular moment in national physical activity discourse, whereby there is '... an accelerating transnationalization of policy norms and practices, the increased mobility of policy techniques and policy makers ... an evolving, experimental policy repertoire, beset by contradictions, as opposed to some fixed blueprint' (Peck and Theodore, 2010). This chapter examines this transnationalisation of policy norms and practices with regard to physical activity policy.

This chapter is informed by a political economy lens and draws on policy studies theories of agenda setting and discourse analysis (Stone, 2002). The year 2014 was selected as the timescale for the analysis as it was a particularly prominent year for physical activity lobbying and policy making, with the publication of two significant Government physical activity documents and two major lobby documents being published. The four documents were chosen for their perceived legitimacy, their large scale and the significant amount of publicity they received. All four documents could reasonably be described as physical activity 'calls to action'. The documents are *Turning the Tide of Inactivity* (UKActive, 2014), *Moving More, Living More: The Physical Activity Olympic and Paralympic Legacy for the Nation* (UK Department of Health, 2014), *Tackling Physical Inactivity: A Co-ordinated Approach* (APCPA, 2014) and *Everybody Active, Every Day: An Evidence-based Approach to Physical Activity* (Public Health England, 2014).

Thematic analysis was to guide the analysis. The initial analysis focused on common themes of contestation in public policy of similarity, difference, continuity, discontinuity, causality and solutions. These themes were then organised into the following narrative presented below.

Continuities and discontinuities

What follows are the most pertinent continuities and discontinuities identified within and between the texts. These themes are important because they frame what is possible and contribute to readers' common sense thinking about physical inactivity.

Similarity and difference

There were five common ideas about the solution to physical inactivity which pervaded the documents in various degrees. First, all the documents mention the economic, social and health outcomes of physical activity, such as physical activity leading to "improved health, but also huge potential social and economic benefits" (UK Government, 2014, p. 4). Second, the documents advocate "cross-sector/multi sector approaches, with joined-up thinking" (All Party Commission, 2014 p. 1). Related to this are other popular ideas of the changes being "nationwide" and "industrial scale" (UK Government, 2014, p. 13). Third, "strong leadership" is advocated (UKActive, 2014, p. 7). Fourth, the need for "evidence based" approaches was emphasised, along with increased monitoring, measurement and evaluation of intervention (Public Health England, 2014, p. 4). Fifth and most prominent was the call for a "change of approach" which needed to be strategic and endorsed by everyone in society (UKActive, 2014, p. 4). Three of the documents (excluding *Tackling Physical Inactivity*) make explicit reference to *The Lancet*'s 2012 Special Issue on physical activity (see Kohl *et al.*, 2012). While *The Lancet* Special Issue was not used in this present analysis, it is apparent that all of these five common ideas mentioned above are present in some form in *The Lancet*'s Special Issue. All of the documents echo the principles of an "ecological approach" to physical activity, whereby the policy solution involves numerous sectors and demands significant change, as distinct from small scale individual programmatic interventions (for a critique of the ecological approach, see Piggin and Bairner, 2014).

Despite the apparent agreement in many aspects of the four documents, there is one instance which highlights an escalation in rhetoric about what is required to make significant population change. This increasingly heightened rhetoric demonstrates that the issue of physical activity has been framed as being of much greater import by Public Health England, than by the earlier UK Government document *Moving More, Living More*, which referred to the supposed legacy from the Olympic Games. It has become apparent that, following the Olympic Games, there has not been a widespread increase in participation, and actually in many cases, participation decreased (Gibson, 2015). More important, however, is the allegation by the All Party Commission on Physical Activity that the UK Government's original vision "does not go far enough" (All Party Commission, 2014, p. 6). In the context of the UK Government having just been involved with the 2012 Olympic Games, a large component of which was the supposed health legacy related the event, to claim that the UK Government did not go far enough is a relatively significant public criticism. Further, two weeks before *Moving More, Living More* was published, UKActive discussed at length the major public health ramifications of physical inactivity, particularly around premature death rates in the UK. It is clear that the importance and size of the problem led Public Health England to produce a significantly more structured and focused publication than *Moving More, Living More*.

A call for revolution

Everybody Active, Every Day was published by Public Health England, the government agency which aims to "protect and improve the nation's health and wellbeing, and reduce health inequalities" (Public Health England, 2015), and is therefore an official authoritative strategy for affecting physical activity. This section considers the nature of the action to be taken. In line with the other documents, calls for large-scale, cross-sector changes, one of the more provocative articulations was references to "change" (UK Government, 2014, p. 4) and in particular, "radical change" (Coe, 2014, p. 14) and "revolution" (Public Health England, 2014, p. 18). This terminology evokes ideas about the fundamental overthrowing of established ways of organising and behaving:

We need to create an appetite for a revolution in physical activity and then light the blue touch paper.

(p. 18)

Social norms can only shift if we can change attitudes radically.

(p. 13)

We need to activate professionals … the media, trade unions, transport, education and business to bring about radical change.

(p. 14)

These claims contain various phrases which illuminate how change will be produced. The first two imply imagery of abrupt, large-scale change to the social order, with their reference to "revolution", "radically" and "light the blue touch paper" for a supposed subsequent 'explosion' of activity. This phrasing has escalated from the earlier UK Department of Health's *Moving More, Living More*, which is rhetorically more modest in its "commitment to promote physical activity across the country's population" (UK Government, 2014, p. 4). Reading the document in its entirety, however, it is clear that while "revolution" is called for, the emphasis is placed upon *other* organisations and groups becoming revolutionary. The reference to creating "an appetite" and "chang[ing] attitudes", along with the aim to "activate professionals" places the onus distinctly upon others. Of course, to a certain extent this is understandable given the disparate groups and individuals involved. However, this also illuminates the perceived level of involvement in the mechanics of the change by Public Health England. That is, Public Health England positions itself as *initiating* the change but not necessarily providing significant resources or legislative support mechanisms.

Despite this emphasis on radical, revolutionary change, there are many implicit challenges to this idea. For example, Public Health England claims it "can help lead the movement for change, but there is no quick fix. It will take long-term promotion of physical activity over months, years and decades" (Public Health England, 2014, p. 13). The revolutionary rhetoric cannot be reconciled with this suggestion of the slow pace of change. Further, other remarks also argue against the idea of radical change. For example, Public Health England claim that "If we want everyone to be active every day, physical activity needs to be made easy, fun and affordable" (Public Health England, 2014, p. 12). This remark implies that while significant change to environment structures might be needed through radical reorganisation, individuals themselves are required to expend little financial cost and little effort. This imperative (or need) places a large onus then, on structural reorganisation. However, there are instances which conflict with this sentiment. For example, at the launch event of *Everybody Active, Every Day*, speaker Sebastian Coe remarked that this "revolutionary" change would "rely on modest adjustments" (Coe, 2014). Similarly in *Everybody Active, Every Day*, remarks are made about the relative small changes that individuals might make:

> Physical activity does not need to be strenuous to be effective. Thirty minutes a day of moderate aerobic activity can be a brisk walk, a swim, or even a spell of gardening.... Each ten-minute bout that gets the heart rate up has a health benefit.
>
> (Public Health England, 2014, p. 10)

Given that the rhetoric of revolution is prominent throughout the documents, the next section investigates the means by which any such change will be produced.

Investment ... or imagination?

The wider context in the UK is that between 2009 and 2015, the UK Government imposed significant public funding cuts to attempt to reduce national debt. The austerity policies would "raise taxes, cut numerous social benefits to millions, shed up to half a million public-sector jobs, cut budgets for government departments, and transfer the onus to create new jobs onto the private sector" (O'Rouke, 2010). Indeed, many cuts have recently been imposed. For example, one of the most prominent recent changes was the dismantling of the School Sport Partnership scheme which had achieved much in terms of ensuring that state school pupils were given opportunities to play sport. Recent research claims that "primary physical education appears to have been a key loser in this policy transition and that a new tier of problems for practice may have unexpectedly been generated" (Mackintosh, 2012, p. 447).

Funding the physical activity revolution was a source of contention throughout the various documents. All of the four documents in this analysis were written in 2014, and were therefore undoubtedly affected by the prevailing economic and political ideology. While funding is not discussed at length in any of the documents, there are statements which imply that despite the aforementioned shared unity in many of the principles for action, the financial implications are a major point of contention. For instance, *Turning the Tide of Physical Inactivity* claims that "There is a disproportionately low spend on programmes to tackle physical inactivity by local authorities compared to other top tier public health concerns"

(UKActive, 2014, p. 8). Similarly, *Tackling Physical Inactivity: A Co-ordinated Approach* states that

> This urgent need also comes at a time of austerity and fiscal constraint. While we recognise that some of the recommendations in this report will have budgetary implications, we also believe that much can be achieved through the reallocation of existing budgets.
>
> (All Party Commission, 2014, p. 6)

In both of these documents therefore, there is lobbying for either new or differently distributed finances. This can be contrasted with remarks by Public Health England, which forthrightly claims that:

> Much of this is not about new investment; it's about maximising the potential of the many assets we already have … and thinking differently about how we commission and plan public services
>
> (Public Health England, 2014, p. 18)

This emphasis on "thinking differently" is repeated elsewhere in the document. For example, "Existing spaces, from forests to school playgrounds, can be used more imaginatively" (Public Health England, 2014, p. 16) and "Re-shaping the world we live in can be done with sensitivity, tapping into and improving existing resources such as canal footpaths, disused railways and river paths" (p. 16). It appears therefore that this revolution would be powered not so much by financial investment but by the ideas, imagination and 'different thinking' of stakeholders involved. Indeed, specific discussions about funding are conspicuous by their relative absence. Basing a revolution on the imagination within the organisations listed above places significant responsibility on certain individuals. For example, a local council physical activity promoter would need to possess both the requisite imagination to implement new ideas, as well as the ability to do so at a time when austerity measures mean that there might well be a *decreased* budget.

Copying Finland

Finland is prominent in both *Tacking Physical Activity* and *Everybody Active, Every Day*. In the former, Finnish policy from 40 years ago to the present day is praised for its effects on physical activity rates and life expectancy (All Party Commission, 2014). In the latter, Finland is repeatedly mentioned as an archetypal nation that is "far more active after a long term, nationwide, locally-based campaign to encourage physical activity across the life course" (Public Health England, 2014, p. 10). Financial implications are downplayed by Public Health England who claim that "The experience in Finland and elsewhere shows that effectively increasing population levels of physical activity involves two common factors: persistence and collaboration" (p. 11).

Despite the use of this energising rhetoric, it is germane to interrogate this narrative alongside other confounding evidence. First, the economic and social conditions of the UK in 2014 and Finland in the 1976 are vastly different. Second and more importantly, the case study which Public Health England relies upon to tell the story of Finland actually makes claims which do not align with the focus on the "imagination" proposed by Public Health England. For example Vuori *et al.* (2004) note that "Participation in sports takes place at the local level. Therefore, municipalities and local organizations are the primary partners to be supported and strengthened" (Vuori *et al.*, 2004, p. 342). However it is clear that UK municipalities have faced and continue to face significant funding cuts. Since 2012, English "culture and leisure services have been subject to budget reductions, [and] there has been a significant increase in the closure or decommissioning of front line services" (Chief Cultural and Leisure Officers Association, 2015). These recent changes conflicts with Vuori *et al.*'s description of the Finnish situation, whereby:

> the Ministry of Education decided to direct, over a five-year period, a major proportion of state support for the construction and maintenance of sites for physical activity to sites serving ordinary people in their daily environments.... This change in funding policy led to increased opportunities for regular physical activity in Finns' daily living environments.
>
> (Vuori *et al.*, 2004, p. 334)

Recent research notes the emphasis in Finnish policy on both the individual and the environment:

> As compared with the Swedish programme, more is written about these social or living conditions and therefore a greater responsibility is placed on the government regarding improving health ... In this sense, the Finnish policy is more social democratic in its approach.
>
> (Vallgårda, 2011, p. 9)

Echoing this, Vehmas noted various significant structural determinants contribute to the Finnish sportive tradition, including the general level of welfare, the number of facilities, and gender equality, and significant school sport (Vehmas, 2011). The UK does not fare particularly well by comparison. Despite this, Vehmas concluded that "Finland is a case of contradiction in physical activity participation: a sportive nation with a lot of (health-related) symptoms of inactive life style". There is a tension therefore, between using Finland as an example to follow in the UK, while also downplaying significant structural change and promoting 'imagination'. Using Nordic sports movement and clubs as one example, Bairner notes these have

> been assisted greatly in their efforts by public support, not least financial, for the provision of facilities. It is doubtful if this would have been possible without the high levels of taxation that were long identified with the social democratic project.

> (2010, p. 736)

Moreover, other research suggests that public policy makers should be cautious about relying on Finland as an exemplar. A recent study "confirmed previous results of cross-sectional studies from several countries that physical activity declines dramatically during youth" (Telema and Yang, 2000, p. 1621). Another study concluded that while youth leisure time physical activity had increased over 30 years, the authors did not consider the trend in Finland to be wholly positive "as it implies increased differences between social classes in leisure time activity" (Laakso *et al.*, 2008, p. 151). Arguably this is already true of the UK according to commentators on what was intended to be the legacy of the 2012 London Olympic Games.

Analysis

UK physical activity promoters have produced an array of lobby documents which share various themes. Stakeholders who are targeted by these calls to action will need to incur significant financial costs themselves to implement change. In their current form, the proposals do not commit to either legislation or resource allocation to make radical change occur. This case study involved a comparative policy analysis of four 'calls to action' created in the UK. Many of these documents recommend that large-scale societal change is needed to avoid the grave consequences of physical inactivity. However, there are also significant differences regarding how change is funded and what the manifestations of these changes are. In particular, the most authoritative document, *EveryBody Active, Every Day*, foregrounds the application of a Finnish physical activity template to the UK. This present analysis demonstrates that, while it is important to reflect on practices elsewhere, it is seldom possible to translate policies from one society to another with very different sociocultural contexts. This is further complicated with regard to the relative lack of financial input to influence this revolution. This analysis concludes by arguing that if significant increases in population-wide physical activity are to be realised, changes in both legislation and funding streams are also required. Otherwise, there is a danger that this will simply be an imagined revolution.

Around both developed and developing nations, there is an increasing impetus to promote physical activity in order to have healthy nations. By analysing the agendas and discourse operating in the UK physical activity policy context, we wanted to first trace the emerging ideas which guide policy decisions, and second, evaluate the extent to which these ideas were coherent. By illuminating the gaps between policy rhetoric (discourse) and reality, the ideas presented here should allow policy makers to be more circumspect with regard to the possibilities of policy interventions. With a social problem of this scale, policy makers need to be both more cautious when reading about, and more sceptical when writing about societal revolutions, stakeholder imaginations and replicable nations. UK physical activity promoters have produced an array of lobby documents which share various themes. Stakeholders who are targeted by these calls to action will need to incur significant financial costs themselves to implement change.

There is much consensus in the various calls to action regarding health, social and economic rationales for physical activity promotion, as well as claims that changes need to be cross-sector, nationwide, industrial scale and evidence-based. Another common element is the praising and desire to learn from the Finnish health policy. However, the analysis demonstrates that, unlike the Finnish exemplar referred to, calls for radical, revolutionary change are not linked with either significant legislative changes or significant investment. In their current form, the UK proposals do not commit to produce legislation or funding to accompany radical change.

Case study 2: the World Health Organisation Strategy for Physical Activity

In the middle of 2018, the World Health Organisation launched the *Global Action Plan on Physical Activity 2018–2030* (WHO, 2018a). Its mission is

> to ensure that all people have access to safe and enabling environments and to diverse opportunities to be physically active in their daily lives, as a means of improving individual and community health and contributing to the social, cultural and economic development of all nations.

(WHO, 2018a, p. 8)

Its target is a "15% relative reduction in the global prevalence of physical inactivity in adults and in adolescents by 2030" (WHO, 2018a, p. 8). The creation of the strategy involved stages of public and stakeholder consultation with the resulting 101-page document incorporating a wide variety of rationalities for promoting physical activity and ideas for implementation 'at scale'. In fact, 'scale' is a term that is repeated often in the policy, signifying a concern for the need to widen the distribution of physical activity programmes. The policy is perhaps the most sophisticated physical activity programme ever produced; its complexity comes from the wide range of settings, motives and ideas for endorsing physical activity. For example, a straight-forward content analysis of the document reveals the following benefits of physical activity, all mentioned at least once in the document, in order of appearance:

- help prevent and treat noncommunicable diseases (NCDs) such as

    - heart disease,
    - stroke,
    - diabetes,
    - breast cancer,
    - colon cancer,

- helps to prevent

    - hypertension,
    - overweight,
    - obesity,

- improve

    - mental health,
    - quality of life,
    - well-being,

- societies can generate additional returns on investment,

    - reduced use of fossil fuels,
    - cleaner air (reducing the numbers of deaths and illnesses from air pollution),
    - less congested roads,
    - safer roads,

- key driver of

    - tourism,
    - employment,
    - infrastructure,

- can also help in humanitarian programmes,
- fostering community development,
- social integration,
- important for
  - early childhood,
  - healthy growth and development in children and adolescents,
  - providing physical and health literacy for long-lasting healthy, active lifestyles,
  - greater ability to concentrate and improved cognitive function, thereby resulting in better academic outcomes,
  - maintain physical health,
  - mental health,
  - social health,

- enable healthy ageing,
- a means to increase rates of rehabilitation and recovery,
- achievement of the 2030 Agenda for Sustainable Development,
- good health and well-being,
- ending all forms of malnutrition,
- quality education – motor skills, and positive attitudes and habits,
- gender equality – ending discrimination, and aiming to enable women and girls to develop transferable skills that enable a more self-reliant life and lead to income-generating activities as well as economic participation,
- decent work and economic growth,
- industry, innovation and infrastructure,
- reduced inequalities,
- sustainable cities and communities,
- responsible production and consumption,
- climate action,
- life on land,
- peace, justice and strong institutions,
- partnerships,
- delay in the onset of dementia,
- can provide enjoyment,
- can also contribute in emergency and crisis situations as part of humanitarian programmes,
- can contribute to increased productivity,
- reduction in injuries,
- reduction in absenteeism,
- prevent falls,
- Ending Childhood Obesity,

- Action for Road Safety,
- Women's, Children and Adolescents' Health,
- Newborn Action Plan to End Preventable Deaths,
- Disability Action Plan,
- Action on Nutrition,
- individual well-being,
- family well-being,
- community well-being,
- social, economic, environmental co-benefit,
- promote and safeguard the rights of all people, of all ages, to have equitable access to safe places and spaces, in their cities and communities,
- highly connected neighbourhoods,
- the use of public transport,
- safe, universal and equitable access by people of all ages and abilities,
- reduce risk for the most vulnerable road users,
- promote public amenities, schools, health care, sports and recreation facilities, workplaces and social housing that are designed to enable occupants and visitors,
- community and patient involvement,
- increase the opportunities for physical activity in the least active groups, as identified by each country, such as girls, women, older adults, rural and indigenous communities, and vulnerable or marginalised populations.

This enormous, multifarious list, ranging from the provision of enjoyment, the support of peace and justice, to the achievement of the 2030 Agenda for Sustainable Development, shows how wide the proposed benefits for physical activity are. At times there is some overreach with some of the goals, such as the inclusion of the development goal of "Zero Hunger" being connected with obesity and overweight, with the explanation that "Overweight and obesity are forms of malnutrition" (p. 52). There is some imprecision too, with the quote that "Physical activity is a core risk factor for NCDs" (p. 53). However, overall, the policy is totalising, in that most physical spaces and places of human life (work, leisure, education, and transport) are encapsulated within it. With such totality, the next question for analysis is how are these goals to be achieved?

There are some dominant frameworks for action throughout the policy. These include systems thinking – "a strategic combination of 'upstream' policy actions aimed at improving the social, cultural, economic and environmental factors ... combined with 'downstream', individually focused (educational and informational) approaches" (p. 8). Various other themes that are deployed include a call for a "paradigm shift" (p. 6), the blaming of "technology" (p. 7) for negatively affecting physical activity rates –

while at the same time promoting the idea of "opportunities for digital innovations to promote and support people of all ages to be more active" (p. 7), the emphasis on health as a human right, and the lament that "progress to increase physical activity has been slow" (p. 6). Overall, though, the emphasis is on multiple opportunities, benefits, sectors, settings, domains and departments. In fact, the idea of something having multiple aspects to it arises 44 times within the policy. There are so many justifications and reasons for physical activity promotion, it becomes clear that the physical activity discourse can now be attached to any policy domain.

Analysis: the proportional universality conundrum of physical activity policy

One of the guiding principles of the entire policy is that of proportional universality – the idea the implementation should focus on "*the greatest efforts directed towards the least active populations*" (WHO, 2018a, p. 11, italics added). It is at least interesting to note that one of the *previous* WHO plans on physical activity contained the principle that "Priority should be given to activities that have a positive impact on the *poorest population groups and communities*" (WHO, 2004, p. 5, italics added). From 2018, directing "the greatest efforts towards the least active populations" results in a conundrum for policy implementers. This is because, in many countries, the least active societies are often the most advanced, long-living societies. This section problematises the principle of *proportional universality* as it applies to *physical activity*. The analysis is guided by the idea that physical activity rates in and of themselves may be too simplistic a measure on which to base which policy interventions. Indeed, on pages 6 and 7 of the WHO policy it is noted that "*As countries develop economically, levels of inactivity increase*" (italics added). If we assume that the least active nations have the most to gain from increasing amounts of physical activity (as denoted by the wide list of benefits noted in the list above – not simply being more active), this means that most of the attention would regularly be directed to often more economically wealthy societies with generally a high quality of life and associated long life expectancies. Statistics from various nations highlight this conundrum. World Health Organisation (2018b) statistics on the "Prevalence of insufficient physical activity among adults" aged 18+ years (as a percentage) are contrasted with 2011 WHO data (2013) on countries' life expectancies in Table 5.1.

While the list in Table 5.1 is not exhaustive, it does connote the difficulty in appraising the level of need in any given country. This makes for difficult decisions in terms of deployment of resources (especially considering that the 2012 *Lancet* Special Issue on physical activity was so concerned with avoiding premature death). Following the logic of proportional universality, should

Table 5.1 Various national activity levels compared with life expectancies

Country	Inactivity level (%)	Life expectancy (in years)
Mozambique	5.6	53
Uganda	5.5	56
Tanzania	6.5	59
Vanuatu	8.0	72
Togo	9.8	56
Belarus	14.1	71
Brazil	47.0	74
Malaysia	38.8	74
USA	40.0	79
Portugal	43.1	80
Australia	30.4	82
Saudi Arabia	53.1	75
Kuwait	67.0	80
Italy	41.4	82

Italy be targeted, or should Uganda? Australia or Tanzania? Other factors could be considered, such as overall population (and therefore overall suffering from inactivity). In any case, utilitarian policy making would argue for the *greatest good* for the greatest number, and if a health promoter was limited to *only* promote physical activity, with "the greatest efforts directed towards the least active populations", then the answer would counter-intuitively be that the greatest efforts should go towards advanced, relatively liberal societies, such as Italy, Australia and Kuwait. This is certainly very different from the direction of the 2004 WHO policy, which focused on the poorest populations groups and communities.

Also, depending on how any given population is divided up, directing the greatest efforts towards the least active populations might necessarily mean focusing mainly on older populations. Some figures bear this out. In 2008 in England, 52 per cent of men and 34 per cent of women aged 16–24 years met government guidelines for physical activity, while only 8 per cent of men and 5 per cent of women aged 75+ years did (Joint Health Surveys Unit, 2010).

Of course, a health promoter might mention that the statistics are aggregated and do not account for specific target groups in any one country. However, given the rhetoric of the policy about promoting *systems* and the call to member states to "promote the different ways *everyone* can increase physical activity and reduce sedentary behaviour" (p. 63, italics added), there remains a confounding correlation in many countries between the overall low levels of activity and high life expectancies. Also, it is interesting that the WHO policy does not emphasise the avoidance of premature death as an explicit rationality. This appears to be the case as it has been both connoted (or given a proxy) by the discussion of diseases such as cancer, as well as being discursively subsumed by the great variety of physical activity promotion justifications listed earlier.

The conundrum of a paradigm shift vs culturally appropriate activities

The WHO plan on physical activity begins by calling for "the need for a whole-of-society response to *achieve a paradigm shift* in both supporting and valuing all people being regularly active, according to ability and across the life course" (p. 6, italics added). The idea of paradigm shifts (elsewhere phrased in policy claims as 'revolutionary' and 'radical' thinking as noted earlier in this chapter) is more than a simple rhetorical device. Given the documented and lamented lack of progress on physical activity rates around the world, the WHO policy explicitly calls for significant changes to takes place. While this is a laudable goal, it must be placed in context with other values mentioned in the document. In the plan to "create active societies" (p. 66), the WHO suggest there is a need to "provide free access to enjoyable and affordable, socially- and *culturally appropriate experiences of physical activity"* (p. 66, italics added). When contrasted with a paradigm shift, the idea of promoting *culturally appropriate* activities might inadvertently exclude potentially transformative activities. One need only think of activities such as skateboarding, snowboarding, surfing. All of these activities at one time were *not* culturally appropriate. However, over time, these activities have become more tolerated and more widely accepted. The same can be said of perceived dangerous sports, or sports that might be perceived to promote harm, such as boxing and martial arts in prisons. For example, recently in the UK there was debate over whether such activities should be taught in prisons (Helm, 2018). Another issue with promoting what is culturally appropriate might mean endorsing communities which have restrictive rules about what physical activities women and men are permitted to do in public spaces, and whether different groups are allowed to participate together. If the physical inactivity problem is as serious as it is framed in the policy, perhaps a greater call would be for people to confront and transcend physical activity norms within their given cultures if they exclude or marginalise individuals' desires to be active.

Conclusion

There is little documented evidence of the successful energising of an entire country (or planet) to become more active and continue such activity over a sustained period. However, both at a national and supra-national level, concerted efforts are being made to do so. Policy and advocacy documents alike call for revolutions, radical changes and paradigm shifts to physical activity changes at a large scale. The deployment of these calls to action is certainly optimistic and it is assumed here that they are made by benevolent advocates. However, these claims must be contrasted with other values within documents which might inadvertently work against significant, radical change.

References

All Party Commission on Physical Activity [APCPA] (2014). *Tackling Physical Inactivity: A Co-ordinated Approach.* England, UK: APCPA.

Bailey, R., Hillman, C., Arent, S. and Petipas, A. (2013). Physical activity: An underestimated investment in human capital. *Journal of Physical Activity and Health, 10,* 289–308.

Bairner, A. (2010). What's Scandinavian about Scandinavian sport? *Sport in Society: Cultures, Commerce, Media, Politics, 13*(4), 734–743.

Chief Cultural and Leisure Officers Association (2015). Financial Settlements for Culture & Leisure 15/16 and beyond. Retrieved from www.cloa.org.uk/current-issues/key-issues/186-financial-settlements-for-culture-a-leisure-1516-and-beyond

Coe, S. (2014, 23 October). Speech at Launch of EveryBody Active, Every Day. Public Health England. London.

Engeli, I. and Allison, C.R. (eds) (2014). *Comparative Policy Studies: Conceptual and Methodological Challenges.* Basingstoke: Palgrave Macmillan.

Gibson, O. (2015, 11 June). Olympic legacy ends in lethargy as sporting participation plummets. *Guardian.*

Helm, T. (2018). Government rejects proposal to teach boxing in prisons. Retrieved from www.theguardian.com/society/2018/jul/07/prisons-reform-boxing-martial-arts-phillip-lee

Joint Health Surveys Unit (2010). *Health Survey for England 2008: Physical Activity and Fitness.* Leeds, UK: The NHS Information Centre.

Kohl, H.W., Craig, C.L., Lambert, E.V., Inoue, S., Alkandari, J.R., Leetongin, G. and Kahlmeier, S., for the Lancet Physical Activity Series Working Group (2012). The pandemic of physical inactivity: Global action for public health. *The Lancet, 380*(9838), 294–305.

Laakso, L., Telema, R., Nupponen, H., Rimpelä, A. and Pere, L. (2008). Trends in leisure time physical activity among young people in Finland, 1977–2007. *European Physical Education Review, 14*(2), 139–155.

Mackintosh, C. (2012). Dismantling the school sport partnership infrastructure: findings from a survey of physical education and school sport practitioners, Education 3–13. *International Journal of Primary, Elementary and Early Years Education, 42*(4), 432–449.

O'Rouke, B. (2010). Britain announces sweeping austerity measures. *Radio Free Europe.* Retrieved from www.rferl.org/a/Britain_Announces_Sweeping_Austerity_Measures/2196108.html

Peck, J. and Theodore, N. (2010). Mobilizing policy: Models, methods, and mutations. *Geoforum, 41*(2), 169–174.

Piggin, J. and Bairner, A. (2014). The global physical inactivity pandemic: An analysis of knowledge production. *Sport, Education and Society, 21*(2), 131–147.

Public Health England (2014). *Everybody Active, Every Day: An Evidence-based Approach to Physical Activity.* London, UK: Public Health England.

Public Health England (2015). About us. Retrieved from www.gov.uk/government/organisations/public-health-england/about.

Stone, D. (2002). *Policy Paradox: The Art of Political Decision Making.* New York: W.W. Norton.

Telema, R. and Yang, X. (2000). Decline of physical activity from youth to young adulthood in Finland. *Medicine and Science in Sport and Exercise, 32,* 1617–1622.

UKActive (2014). Turning the tide of inactivity. UKActive. Retrieved from www.ukactive.com/turningthetide

UK Government (2014). *Moving More, Living More: The Physical Activity Olympic and Paralympic Legacy for the Nation.* UK Government.

Vallgårda, S. (2007). Public health policies: A Scandinavian model? *Scandinavian Journal of Public Health, 35*(2), 205–211.

Vallgårda, S. (2011). Addressing individual behaviours and living conditions: Four Nordic public health policies. *Scandinavian Journal of Public Health, 39,* 6–10.

Vehmas, H. (2011, 5 October). Why do we really rank on top? Socio-cultural interpretations about sport participation in Finland. Paper presented at the *Play the Game Conference*, Cologne.

Vuori, I., Lankenau, B. and Pratt, M. (2004). Physical activity policy and program development: The experience in Finland. *Public Health Reports, 119,* 331–345.

WHO (2004). *Global Strategy on Diet, Physical Activity and Health.* Geneva: World Health Organisation.

WHO (2013). World health statistics, 2013. Retrieved from www.who.int/gho/publications/world_health_statistics/EN_WHS2013_Full.pdf

WHO (2018a). *Global Action Plan on Physical Activity 2018–2030: More Active People for a Healthier World.* Geneva: World Health Organisation.

WHO (2018b). Prevalence of insufficient physical activity among adults. Data by country. Retrieved from http://apps.who.int/gho/data/node.main.A893?lang=en

6 Physical activity and the politics of junk food

Analyses of corporations will always be slanted by one's pre-existing perspective on the motivations of corporations. On one hand there is the pluralist view of corporations, which assumes that corporate entities are a legitimate interest group in a relatively open political framework and should therefore be allowed as much access to decision-making processes and target markets as they endeavour to attain. The thinking of pluralists is that constraining or curtailing the activities of legal entities is problematic, since they have legal rights and to interfere might hinder economic development. On the other hand, a political economy perspective posits that corporations and their ideas dominate large parts of economic and political life unfairly. This perspective assumes that they can contribute to defining the political agenda because of their economic resources and access to decision-making processes which other groups do not have access to (Blowers, 1983). Therefore they can create systems that benefit themselves, possibly to the detriment of the wider society and vulnerable groups, as well as the environment. The externalisation of harms and costs by corporations to others is a significant criticism of corporations.

In recent decades there has been growing suspicion about engaging with corporations to achieve health outcomes. Criticism has focused on the lobbying power of corporations, exploitative labour practices and destructive environmental impacts, all of which are conducted through corporations' legal obligation to maximise profit (Piggin, 2015). A focus of criticism surrounds the deleterious effects on human health from food and drink products emblazoned with 'health' branding despite being ultra-processed. (Piggin *et al.*, 2017). Much of this anti-corporate narrative can be linked to attacks on the neo-liberal agenda and its perceived negative impact on communities' and individuals' health.

An editorial in the *Journal of Public Health* referred to corporations as "vectors of disease" (2011, p. 2). Companies linking their products with sport and physical activity have also faced criticism about their behaviour.

Collin and MacKenzie (2006) described sponsorship of the English Football Association by McDonald's and Pepsi as "inappropriate ... and highly questionable" (p. 1964). Further, they believed the goal of the 2012 London Olympic Games; "to inspire sporting activity and achievement and foster a healthy and active nation [is] difficult to reconcile with McDonald's and Coca-Cola as official sponsors" (p. 1964). By using phrases such as "may be sabotaged", "highly questionable" and "difficult to reconcile" the authors frame corporate involvement as self-evidently problematic. Of course, it is not only food and drink companies that have a vested interest in sport and physical activity promotion, as will be explored in upcoming chapters.

Due to perceptions of a growing obesity issue, claimed government budgetary pressures and limited intervention effects, corporations have increasingly been framed as 'partners' in public health. Around the world, governments, governing bodies and corporations are collaborating for health promotion. The World Health Organisation (WHO) has encouraged cooperation with the private sector for the past two decades. In their 2004 Global Strategy for Physical Activity, the WHO embraced the supposed transformative potential of companies:

> The private sector can be a significant player in promoting healthy diets and physical activity.... All [businesses] could become partners with governments and nongovernmental organizations in implementing measures aimed at sending positive and consistent messages to facilitate and enable integrated efforts to encourage healthy eating and physical activity. Because many companies operate globally, international collaboration is crucial.
>
> (WHO, 2004, p. 13)

Similarly, the 2018 Global Strategy for Physical Activity also mentions the importance of the private sector being "committed to improving the health of employees, their families and communities" (WHO, 2018, p. 24). The global reach and large marketing budgets of multinational corporations are worth discussing. In neo-liberal Western societies particularly, they reach into many aspects of modern life, from supermarket shelves to event sponsorship and mainstream advertising campaigns. Andrew Lansley, the former British Secretary of State for Health, wrote about the unique power of the business sector (while arguably being incorrect about 'many' current corporate practices):

> Businesses have both the technical expertise to make healthier products and the marketing expertise to influence purchasing habits. If the

full strength of these skills can be directed towards activities to encourage and enable people to make healthier choices – as many responsible businesses do already – the benefits could be great.

(Lansley, 2011, p. 2)

The recent and ongoing UK "Change4Life" health promotion campaign involved significant corporate 'cooperation', whereby the UK Department of Health formalised promotional arrangement with many companies. The justification for doing so was that "many of these brands can talk to our audience in ways that we can't – and we can use this to help influence people's behaviour" (Change4Life, 2009). Of course, this decision attracted criticism from a *Lancet* editorial for using corporate sponsors to help fund the Change4Life health campaign:

> It beggars belief that the government has decided to allow sponsorship by commercial companies … [including] PepsiCo and Kellogg's – the makers of the very products that contribute to obesity.

(*The Lancet*, 2009, p. 96)

Similar practices can be seen in Canada. In 2010 in Canada, Kelly Murumets, the CEO of the government-sponsored 'ParticipACTION' brand, promoted the *necessity* and *inevitability* of public–private partnerships in sport and physical activity:

> we have witnessed an increased *need* for partnerships between private companies and the sport and physical activity sector overall. Given the current scarcity of government resources and the potential benefits to both partners, it seems that partnerships are *not only here to stay*, but that they can advance our common interest: to increase the health and physical activity of a population that is increasingly at risk from its sedentary lifestyle.

(ParticipACTION, 2010, p. 2, italics added)

This justification was also echoed in the book *Public–Private Partnerships in Physical Activity and Sport*, where O'Reilly and Brunette (2013) wrote that "in the world of sport and physical activity, developing partnerships makes sense as a way to pool scarce resources" (p. 14). The ParticipACTION *Partnership Protocol* (2010) does discuss potential risks of partnerships, and suggests to not-for-profit organisations (NFPs) that "the corporate 'match' must be compatible with your values, goals and branding. Safeguard your organization's credibility and reputation: *stay true to who you are*" (p. 6, italics added). Contrarily, two pages later NFPs are encouraged to "Be flexible to the needs of your partner..." (p. 8). Further, in a brief section on "acknowledging and managing risk", NFPs are instructed to "Consider the risks and rewards of each potential partner and understand the implications of working with that organization" (p. 8). NFPs are encouraged to consider if the partnership could:

> prevent other partnerships or harm your organization's potential activities in the future. If the controversy is unwarranted, consider how best to overcome opposing viewpoints and be prepared to defend these viewpoints in the public domain when challenged.

(p. 8)

It is apparent the ParticipACTION group was conscious of the potential mismatches but there were no apparent practical examples of what types of partnerships might be inappropriate for NFPs. Given that most consumer brands endorse the vague values of 'health, wellbeing and fitness', this allows for virtually any corporation to match with an NFP seeking assistance. Further, there was no discussion of what the implications might be of inappropriate partnerships.

The protocol culminates in advising NFPs to consider creating "a crisis management plan" to handle any possible large-scale objections to the partnership. This plan would outline key messages and Q&As, and specify (and educate) "a potential spokesperson to counter negative perceptions, internally or externally" (p. 9). And here can be seen one of the problems with partnership logic. While NFP-sport and physical activity organisations are encouraged to counter negative perceptions (of sponsors), there is insufficient attention given to the possibility that "negative perceptions of a corporate sponsor" are fair, reasonable and justified.

The production politics of the ParticipACTION document is telling. Members of the Steering Committee included (but were not limited to): the president of TrojanOne (a marketing company whose clients include Coca Cola), the Vice President of Corporate Affairs for Kellogg, and the Director of Public Affairs and Communications for Coca-Cola Canada. While there were various steps involved in the production of the document, some were curiously oriented towards what would reasonably be considered corporate interests. Corporate sponsorship of sport and physical activity in this case was framed as both inevitable and necessary by lobbyists who have a direct interest in increasing corporate sponsorship of sport and physical activity.

Whether it is the World Health Organisation, the UK Department of Health, or the Canadian ParticipACTION programme, the discourse of positive partnerships is inherently political, and troubling for those who are wary of the potentially detrimental effects of ultra-processed, energy-dense, nutrient-poor food-like products, or other products which are detrimental to health. It raises serious questions about the place of corporations in physical activity promotion and sport provision (for both children and adults). Various academic analyses have cast a critical view on these practices. Accusations of creeping privatisation and contrived philanthropy (Boyles, 2005; Powell, 2018) have been levied at the sports world and education settings for the last two decades. The rhetoric is intensifying, as collusion, inappropriate marketing practices and dubious intervention effects are being exposed by researchers and health advocates around the world.

Hemingway (2005) suggests corporate social responsibility (CSR) practices exist "for the corporation to be seen to be taking its social responsibilities seriously ... regardless of whether this is actually occurring in practice" (p. 233). Humphreys and Brown (2008) call these practices "branding and damage limitation strategies" (p. 404). The supposed logic of these strategies is that the corporations benefit by *appearing* altruistic and benevolent. Wagner, Lutz and Weitz (2009) mention various citizen and community organisation-created critiques "have all revealed more and more company practices that appear socially *irresponsible"* (p. 77, italics added). These critiques of corporate hypocrisy allow the narrative of corporate villains to emerge. That is, corporations are framed as unscrupulous institutions existing only in order to generate profit.

A 'scandal' that exemplifies the scepticism about corporate involvement in sport and health promotion was Cadbury UK's 2003 'Get Active Scheme', which encouraged children and schools to collect tokens from chocolate bars which could be exchanged for school sports equipment. The Food Commission, a UK healthy food campaigning charity called the scheme "absurd" and "contradictory", suggesting that if children ate all the promotional bars they would be consuming nearly two million kilos of fat, and that one set of volleyball posts and nets would require tokens from 5,440 bars (Food Commission, 2003).

This narrative of the health-damaging (as opposed to health-promoting) corporation also informs health literature. For example, in the *Journal of Health Communication*, Rudd, Goldberg and Dietz (1999) state that "public health messages are outnumbered by many commercial sector interests that promote products and activities with unhealthful consequences" (p. 38). In the same journal Berry, McCarville and Rhodes (2008) describe "competing messages" and suggest that "efforts to encourage active living ... may be sabotaged by extensive commercial efforts to promote automobile use and sedentary lifestyles" (p. 170). They also argue that in many instances "sophisticated public health messages provide the only viable alternative to the pervasive commercials *selling untoward health*" (p. 38, italics added).

While academics critique corporate involvement in health promotion, some scholars and scholarly societies have been on the receiving end of criticism. In 2015, de Sá wrote a scathing critique of Coca Cola's sponsorship of the International Society of Physical Activity and Health's conference. He said the conference:

> in Brazil has been sponsored by an organisation [Coca Cola] whose policies, practices, or products conflict with those of public health. The sponsorship was not only financial; Coca Cola was everywhere at side meetings, in the sponsors' hall, giving away its products and propaganda. At a time when sweetened soft drinks are recognised by independent organisations as a major cause of the present uncontrolled obesity pandemic, which notably affects children and developing countries, such as China, India – and Brazil, this is worrying.
>
> (de Sá, 2015)

Academia is implicated in another way too – through its teaching. Regarding courses in sport studies, health and nutrition, some important issues arise for future practice. How should corporations be framed to students who might soon be managers, nutritionists or health consultants within corporations? Writing in the *American Journal of Public Health*, Wiist (2006) proposed that public health curricula should include a focus on "the Corporation as a Fundamental Structural Cause of Disease" (p. 1370).

And so, what is to be done? Should all manner of companies be encouraged to promote physical activity through CSR campaigns? Or, should corporations' massive lobbying capability, history of exploitative labour practices and destructive environmental impacts, all of which are conducted through corporations' legal obligation to focus solely on maximising profit, exclude them from contention as potential sources of health/physical activity promotion? This chapter critiques the practices of a variety of corporations which have claimed to promote health through physical activity promotion, at the same time as promoting their products to young people.

Of course, a variety of defences are available to combat such opposition. First, critics of such programmes do not tend to consider the potentially positive contribution companies could make to physical activity promotion. Second, programmes tend to have numerous financial supporters. A cursory examination of the 2013 Change4Life website revealed that, aside from PepsiCo and Kellogg's, 69 other organisations supported the programme (so that it was not solely a Pepsi and Kellogg's partnership).

Third, sweepingly naming companies as "the makers of the very products that contribute to obesity" neglects the 'healthy' products the companies do offer to the market. Such defences might not appease critics of CSR programmes who argue that all companies involved only want to benefit commercially.

Critics of overbearing corporate interest use several rhetorical devices themselves to frame the involvement of corporations. Claiming corporate greed as the 'real' reason behind supposed benevolent acts is a popular plot-line in the health promotion narrative. This villain narrative is also prominent in newspaper synopses of the Change4Life campaign. In a section entitled 'What are the drawbacks?' the health editor in *The Independent* newspaper wrote:

> Companies *exploit* the link with government for their own commercial ends.... Critics fear the Government has been hoodwinked into providing some of the biggest food and drink companies in the land with a gold-plated opportunity to cast their brands in a healthy light. By linking with the Change4Life campaign they automatically show themselves to be on the side of the *good guys*.
>
> (Lawrence, 2009, ¶ 6, italics added)

The claim that businesses 'exploit', 'hoodwink' and try to be perceived as 'good guys', reinforces a villain narrative. That companies would become involved in a campaign such as this because of a genuine concern for the health of a community is dismissed by the logic that organisations are either 'good' or 'bad'.

Similar criticism has been directed towards the UK Government's Public Health Responsibility Deal (PHRD) (UK Department of Health, 2011). The now defunct PHRD encouraged corporations to promote health. Shadow public health minister Diane Abbott totally opposed the policy. While Abbott suggests that 'business' is important, she reinforces the villain narrative by implying that public health initiatives succeed despite corporate interests:

> The truth is that you cannot conflate corporate responsibility with public health. While the government needs to work very closely with business and industry, all the big changes in public health over the last 200 years have been done in the face of huge corporate and commercial interests.
>
> (Quoted in Triggle, 2011)

Conundrums of critiquing corporate involvement in health promotion

There are other elements to the framing of critique. One assumption that authors such as Collin and MacKenzie make (2006; discussed above) is that the London Olympic Games have the ability to inspire sporting participation and achievement. However, there is a plethora of critical literature which shows that such noble goals (and the International Olympic Committee) are themselves couched in socially constructed narratives which produce an unproblematic vision of the positive 'power of sport'. Indeed, if Collin and MacKenzie levied a similarly critical eye upon the IOC and the Olympic Games as some other authors do (see, for instance, Lenskyj, 2002; Cashman, 2006; Culpan and Wigmore, 2010; Kohe, 2010), their apparent simplistic contradiction would be subsumed into a complex political analysis. This asymmetry of criticism against corporations while holding sports organisations as virtuous (despite allegations of corruption and exploitation) might perpetuate the narrative of 'good vs bad' to the detriment of a more nuanced understanding of power relations. Clearly, recent scandals affecting FIFA, the UCI, and the IAAF all highlight that corporations are not alone in being scrutinised for unethical, inappropriate behaviour.

Insight into the discursive conundrum comes from Dorey and McCool (2009) who asked groups of children about how they thought about the effect of the media on their understandings of health. On 'trusting the corporate messenger' the researchers wrote that while participants moved towards a consensus about the hypocrisy, there were also moments of confusion. One child exclaimed:

> Yeah, but, like, it's McDonald's and McDonald's isn't that healthy, but they're trying to get people to like be active and stuff. It's kind of weird.
>
> (Female in Dorey and McCool, 2009, p. 649)

This articulation of the contradiction – that "It's kind of weird" – is demonstrative of how little is known about attitudes of various citizenries about corporate health promotion. An editorial in *The Lancet* about corporate involvement in Change4Life had a similarly puzzled tone when trying to articulate the repercussions:

> So what is the subliminal, or perhaps not so subliminal, take-home message when PepsiCo brings us sports personalities who advocate exercise? If you do exercise, it is OK to drink Pepsi and eat crisps?
>
> (Change4Life brought to you by PepsiCo, 2009, p. 96)

Researchers of policy, lived experiences and politics might examine the processes that occur between corporations and citizens affected by CSR programmes. As well as this, there is space to analyse in more detail what effects occur when changing the messenger of physical activity and health promotion from the state to companies. Also we might consider the tension between the dominant rhetoric discussed in this analysis with the apparent dominant role corporations play in funding national sports organisations (NSOs). Often official NSO literature praises sponsoring corporations for their benevolent contributions to participation initiatives, and coaching programmes.

Several contradictions and tensions exist when considering private sponsorship arrangements of sport and physical activity programmes. First is the perceived tension between company's profit motive (and behaviour) and claimed social responsibility goals. Second is the tension between various state goals, or antagonistic economic drivers which exist between economic motives and health motives. For example, it may be economically beneficial to have more people 'consume' a product, which will result in more tax income for a government. However, if that product is detrimental to health, there will certainly be deleterious health consequences. For example, Doran *et al.* (1996) estimated that in 1989–1990 an average smoker cost the government $203.57, while revenue from tax received totalled an average of $620.56 in the same year. Therefore the authors suggested that the objective of raising revenue from smoking is more of a priority than reducing smoking rates. The third tension is between sport and physical activity organisations' goals (which often claim to promote health) and the products of the corporate brands and products they accept. With this context in mind, what follows is a synopsis of recent concerns about the promotion of physical activity by the companies which are often what are colloquially termed 'junk food' companies.

The English Football Association and corporate partners

The English Football Association, its various offshoot organisations, along with clubs around the country have a variety of sponsorship arrangements with many companies. Many of these are with companies which promote and sell foods which are classified as unhealthy.

While there is no universal categorisation of foods into 'unhealthy' or 'healthy' categories, research has found that consumers do categorise foods according to a good–bad dichotomy based on specific food qualities (Oakes and Slotterback, 2001; Provencher *et al.*, 2008). Research indicates that a diet filled with processed foods, with high amounts of fat, sugar and sodium, can lead to poorer health outcomes than those which do not (Block *et al.*, 2004; Swinburn *et al.*, 2004; Lewis *et al.*, 2005). With specific regard to sport, Carter *et al.* (2013) found that "the sponsorship relationships between sporting organisations and food and beverage brands and companies do not always reinforce either sports-related or more general nutrition recommendations" (p. 2).

Momentum is gathering towards changing the accepted practices at sports events. The World Health Organisation Commission on Ending Childhood Obesity (2016) argued that young people and adults are negatively affected by unhealthy food messages, and recommended that settings where children and adolescents gather, such as sports facilities or events, should be free of marketing of unhealthy foods and sugar-sweetened beverages. However, the English Football Association and its offshoot enterprises maintain many sponsorship arrangements with companies which sell ultra-processed food and drink. For example, in 2018, as well as Coca Cola, McDonald's and Budweiser sponsoring FIFA (the sport's international federation of football associations), the following arrangements occurred at a national level:

- The English Football Association was sponsored by Coca Cola, McDonald's, Budweiser, Lucozade, Mars and Walker's crisps.
- Wembley Stadium was sponsored by Carlsberg, Walker's, Coca Cola and Mars.
- The Premier League was sponsored by Coca Cola, Carling and Cadbury.
- The English Football League was sponsored by Carabao and Irn-Bru.
- The community/youth level of football was sponsored by McDonald's.

There is significant power wielded by sponsors. For example, McDonald's is sponsoring grass-roots football in England, Scotland, Wales and Northern Ireland. McDonald's claim that:

> Over the next 4 years, we're teaming up with the UK Football Associations to provide opportunities for over 500,000 children aged 5–11 to try football for the first time. We'll be delivering 5 million hours of fun, introductory coaching sessions and family events in local communities near you.
>
> (McDonald's, 2019)

Imagery on the McDonald's website shows young children in sports gear branded with McDonald's logos, being taught by coaches with McDonald's logos, surrounded by banners with McDonald's logos. The appropriateness of such brand saturation of young people by a multinational company known for selling a range of ultra-processed food illustrates how problematic such sponsorship arrangements are.

Conscious decisions to begin and sustain these corporate relationships are particularly problematic, and research is emerging to show what these types of relationships can mean in practice. Jane and Gibson (2018) found that Coca Cola's sponsorship of a 'ParkLives' physical activity programme allowed the corporation to target its marketing at children and gain access to health-related policy development networks. This is despite the company's claim it does not directly market to children under 12 years old (Coca Cola, 2018). Research into the policy which led to the provision of food and drink for spectators at the Rio Olympics found that the organisers and sponsors failed to fulfil their self-proclaimed 'social responsibility' of leading people towards healthy choices. Specifically, the failures included that most of the prominent food and drink for spectators was 'ultra-processed', which the Brazilian Ministry of Health recommends avoiding (Piggin *et al.*, 2019). While events such as the Olympic and Paralympic Games are often touted as inspirational ways of leading young people towards more active lives, the practical manifestations of events can be vastly different – as avenues to promote unhealthy food and drink.

Conclusion

Vandevijvere and Swinburn (2015) wrote:

> The marketing of unhealthy food products to children is ... *powerful* because it influences children's food preferences, purchase requests, and consumption. It is *pervasive* because modern marketing ensures that brands engage with children across multiple media platforms. It is *predatory* because it exploits the credulity of children for commercial gain.
>
> (p. 36)

These practical manifestations of marketing campaigns are the eventual result of policy and political decisions about how sport and physical activity should be organised. That companies have identified and exploited opportunities for commercial gain through sport sponsorship, particularly targeting children, should be no surprise. However, the continued promotion of 'partnership' as opposed to 'regulation' of junk food interests in the sport and physical activity domain is a space where there are changes to be made to have less exploitative outcomes for the people involved.

References

Berry, T.R., McCarville, R.E. and Rhodes, R.E. (2008). Getting to know the competition: A content analysis of publicly and corporate funded physical activity advertisements. *Journal of Health Communication, 13*(2), 169–180.

Block, J.P., Scribner, R.A. and DeSalvo, K.B. (2004). Fast food, race/ethnicity, and income. *American Journal of Preventive Medicine, 27*(3), 211–217.

Blowers, A. (1983). Master of fate or victim of circumstance: The exercise of corporate power in environmental policy-making. *Policy and Politics, 11*, 393–415.

Boyles, D.R. (2005). The exploiting business: School-business partnerships, commercialization, and students as critically transitive citizens. In D.R. Boyles (ed.), *Schools or Markets? Commercialism, Privatization, and School-Business Partnerships* (pp. 217–240). Mahwah, NJ: Lawrence Erlbaum.

Carter, M., Signal, L., Edwards, R., Hoek, J. and Maher, A. (2013). Food, fizzy, and football: Promoting unhealthy food and beverages through sport: A New Zealand case study. *BMC Public Health, 13*, 1–7.

Cashman, R. (2006). *The Bitter-sweet Awakening: The Legacy of the Sydney 2000 Olympic Games*. New South Wales, Australia: Walla Walla Press.

Change4Life (2009). Our national partners. Retrieved from www.nhs.uk/Change4Life/Pages/national-partners.aspx

Coca Cola (2018). Responsible marketing. Retrieved from www.cocacolacompany.com/stories/responsible-marketing

Collin, J. and MacKenzie, R. (2006). The World Cup, sport sponsorship, and health. *The Lancet, 367*, 1964–1966.

Culpan, I. and Wigmore, S. (2010). The delivery of Olympism education within a physical education context drawing on critical pedagogy. *International Journal of Sport and Health Sciences, 8*, 67–76.

de Sá, T.H. (2014). Can Coca Cola promote physical activity? *The Lancet, 383*(9934), 2041.

Doran, C.M., Sanson-Fisher, R.W. and Gordon, M. (1996). A cost-benefit analysis of the average smoker: a government perspective. *Australia and New Zealand Journal of Public Health, 20*, 607–611.

Dorey, E. and McCool, J. (2009). The role of the media in influencing children's nutritional perceptions. *Qualitative Health Research, 19*, 645–654.

Food Commission. (2003). Cadbury wants children to eat two million kg of fat – to get fit! *Food Commission*. Retrieved from www.foodcomm.org.uk/parentsjury/cadbury_03.htm

Hemingway, C.A. (2005). Personal values as a catalyst for corporate social entrepreneurship. *Journal of Business Ethics, 60*(3), 233–249.

Humphreys, M. and Brown, A.D. (2008). An analysis of corporate social responsibility at Credit Line: A narrative approach. *Journal of Business Ethics, 80*, 403–418.

Jane, B. and Gibson, K. (2018). Corporate sponsorship of physical activity promotion programmes: Part of the solution or part of the problem? *Journal of Public Health, 40*, 2, 279–288.

Journal of Public Health (2011). Editorial: Public health, corporations and the New Responsibility Deal: Promoting partnerships with vectors of disease? *Journal of Public Health, 33*(1), 2–4.

Kohe, G. (2010). Disrupting the rhetoric of the rings: a critique of Olympic idealism in physical education. *Sport, Education and Society, 15*(4), 479–494.

The Lancet (2009). Change4Life brought to you by PepsiCo (and others). *The Lancet,* 373, 96.

Lansley, A. (2011). Foreword. In *Public Health Responsibility Deal.* London: UK Department of Health.

Lawrence, J. (2009, 2 January). The big question: Can the Government really make us eat less and exercise to become slim? *The Independent.*

Lenskyj, H. (2002). *The Best Olympics Ever? Social Impacts of Sydney 2000.* USA: New York Press.

Lewis, L.B., Sloane, D.C., Nascimento, L.M., Diamant, A.L., Guinyard, J.J., Yancey, A.K. and Flynn, G. (2005). African Americans' access to healthy food options in South Los Angeles restaurants. *American Journal of Public Health, 95*(4), 668–673.

McDonald's (2019). McDonald's Fun Football. Retrieved from www.mcdonalds. com/gb/en-gb/football.html

Oakes, M.E. and Slotterback, C.S. (2001). Judgements of food healthfulness: Food name stereotypes in adults over age 25. *Appetite, 37,* 1–8.

O'Reilly, N. and Brunette, M.K. (2013). *Public–Private Partnerships in Physical Activity and Sport.* USA: Human Kinetics.

ParticipACTION (2010). *The Partnership Protocol. Principles and Approach for Successful Private/ Not-for-Profit Partnerships in Physical Activity and Sport.* Canada.

Piggin, J. (2015). Designed to move? Physical activity lobbying and the politics of productivity. *Health Education Journal, 74*(1), 16–27.

Piggin, J., Tlili, H. and Louzada, B. (2017). How does health policy affect practice at a sport mega event? A study of policy, food and drink at Euro 2016. *International Journal of Sport Policy and Politics, 9*(4), 739–751.

Piggin, J., Souza, D.L., Furtado, S., Milanez, M., Cunha, G., Louzada, B.H., Graeff, B. and Tlili, H. (2019). Do the Olympic Games promote dietary health for spectators? An interdisciplinary study of health promotion through sport. *European Sport Management Quarterly.* doi: 10.1080/16184742.2018.1562484

Powell, D. (2018). Culture jamming the 'corporate assault' on schools and children. *Global Studies of Childhood, 8*(4), 379–391.

Provencher, P., Polivy, J. and Herman, CP. (2008). Perceived healthiness of food: If it's healthy, you can eat more! *Appetite, 52*(2), 340–344.

Rudd, R., Goldberg, J. and Dietz, W. (1999). A five staged model for sustaining a community campaign. *Journal of Health Communication, 4,* 37–48.

Swinburn, B., Caterson, I., Seidell, J. and James, W. (2004). Diet, nutrition and the prevention of excess weight gain and obesity. *Public Health Nutrition, 7*(1A), 123–146.

Triggle, N. (2011). Health groups 'reject responsibility deal' on alcohol. *BBC.* Retrieved from www.bbc.co.uk/news/health-12728629

UK Department of Health (2011). *Public Health Responsibility Deal*. London: UK Department of Health.

Vandevijvere, S. and Swinburn, B. (2015). Getting serious about protecting New Zealand children against unhealthy food marketing. *New Zealand Medical Journal*, 128, 36–40.

Wagner, T., Lutz R.J. and Weitz, B.A. (2009). Corporate hypocrisy: Overcoming the threat of inconsistent corporate social responsibility perceptions. *Journal of Marketing*, *73*, 77–91.

WHO (2004). *Global Strategy on Diet, Physical Activity and Health*. Geneva: World Health Organisation.

WHO (2016). *Commission on Ending Childhood Obesity. Report of the Commission on Ending Childhood Obesity*. Geneva: World Health Organisation.

WHO (2018). *Global Action Plan on Physical Activity 2018–2030: More Active People for a Healthier World*. World Health Organisation, Geneva.

Wiist, W.H. (2006). Proposed additions to public health curricula: the corporation as a fundamental structural cause of disease. *American Journal of Public Health*, *96*(8), 1370–1375.

7 Physical activity and the politics of corporate health promotion

Introduction[1]

As well as traditional state interventions, there are intensifying efforts by a range of non-state actors to motivate people to be more physically active. This chapter examines three aspects of the Nike corporation's involvement with the global and UK discourses of physical activity. First, it examines Nike's involvement in building a theory about physical activity. Second, it considers Nike's alliance with a variety of state, civil society and professional organisations in the process of constructing their 'Designed To Move' lobby document. Third, the chapter examines Nike's attempted construction of a global physical activity 'movement' in association with the UK Physical Activity Commission. By interrogating the political activities of the Nike corporation, we can see how physical activity is deployed to meet specific economic ends.

Nike's lobbying for physical activity

In recent years, Nike has developed connections in the physical activity sphere which eclipsed any traditional sponsorship arrangement. Part of their focus was the production of a physical activity 'movement' called 'Designed To Move' (DTM). The main DTM report was published in September 2012. It was "presented by Nike, The American College of Sports Medicine, The International Council of Science & Physical Education and several other expert organizations" (Nike *et al.*, 2012). It promoted multi-sector approaches to physical activity promotion. It appealed to "change-makers" to intervene because "the world has stopped moving". The launch was accompanied by a melodramatic video, which featured many young children describing what they would do if they could live for five extra years – this supposedly being the extra time they would benefit from by being physically active throughout their lives.

The Human Capital Model

In 2013, an article was published in the Journal of Physical Activity and Health discussing the wide-ranging benefits of physical activity (Bailey *et al.*, 2013). The article proposed the Human Capital Model, which theorised that physical activity can contribute to various forms of capital for an individual, including emotional, financial, individual, intellectual, physical, and social capitals. The Human Capital Model

> suggests not only that physical activity is a key driver of different types of capital formation, but that the capitals in turn influence both physical activity and each other; forming a synergistic feedback network whose whole is greater than the sum of its parts.
>
> (Bailey *et al.*, p. 290)

The article is 'aspirational', though it also shows the power of corporations to become involved in ideas about health promotion. The text surrounding the model suggests the 'Human Capital Model' was not produced by the authors of the article, but by Nike Inc. We might ask, why is Nike, a global sportswear company, interested in publishing a theoretical model in an academic journal? The Acknowledgements section in the article suggests how the model came to be: "In 2010 NIKE, Inc. developed the Human Capital Model, informed by more than 500 pieces of published research, and initiated a multidisciplinary input and validation process with a pool of experts" (p. 302). Notwithstanding the interesting collection of rationalities for promotion of physical activity, the article includes a chart which suggests that *"financial capital"* is *"reliant on all the other Capitals"* (p. 301, italics added).

The flow chart in Figure 7.1 contains many interesting assumptions if one analyses the politics at play. First, there are likely to be many people around the world who have high levels of financial capital without having a significant amount of physical, emotional, individual, intellectual or social capital (see Piggin, 2015). Even a cursory analysis of one's own social network and community (or personal introspection) might provide examples to show the fallacy that financial capital is "reliant on all the other Capitals".

Second, it is readily apparent that many forms of capital depend on possessing or being born into families with financial capital to begin with. The same is true of the wider community one is born into. The advantages and privileges afforded by having access to financial capital are numerous.

Third, the elevation of financial capital to the pinnacle of Figure 7.1 implies that money is the desired outcome to be attained. Framing financial

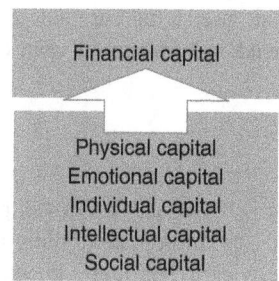

Figure 7.1 Adaptation of flow chart published in the *Journal of Physical Activity and Health*, with copyright to Nike. The associated text claimed that that financial capital is "reliant on all the other capitals" (see Bailey *et al.*, 2013).

capital as the outcome of various forms of capital is perhaps the most overt display of Western neo-liberal thinking articulated in a scholarly journal on physical activity to date. Possessing any or all the forms of capital in the model is simply a way of acquiring something else – money. Of course, Nike is obligated to make a profit for its shareholders, but we need to recall what a singular focus on increasing financial capital can lead to. In 2005, Nike's own report of the factories that made its shoes and clothing admitted "excessively long work weeks, wrong wage calculations, verbal abuse, curbs on toilet visits" and a pervasive culture of exploitation (see Nike, 2005). Nike's admission of worker abuses shows how those with financial capital can exploit those without.

Fourth, nowhere in the article is any evidence provided for the claim: "Financial capital [is] reliant on all the other Capitals". It is written simply as a truism. The idea of being born into families or societies of great wealth is absent from the model and its explanation.

Fifth, a critical reader might ask, to whom do the authors encourage this financial capital to belong? Bailey *et al.* emphasise individual financial capital accumulation by "highlight[ing] the ways in which engagement in physical activity can act as an asset that enhances career and financial success" (p. 301). Readers might ask, is the accumulation of financial capital a worthy goal, especially when there are such stark differences in the current global distribution of wealth?

The Human Capital Model gained traction by virtue of being replicated by the UK All Party Commission on Physical Activity (APCPA), an unofficial government taskforce aiming to address the physical inactivity pandemic. In turn, the APCPA was commended by a UK Government policy document for advancing the physical activity agenda. While the specific flow chart was not referenced, it is certainly an interesting case that a corporation was able to have published in an academic journal its own conception of how resources flow in society.

Designed To Move

Closely related to the Human Capital Model was 'Designed To Move', published in September 2012, mentioned earlier. The introduction boldly proclaimed a crisis – "the world has stopped moving". The lobby document would advocate for a multisectoral approach to physical activity promotion, aiming at 'changemakers' to make people around the world more physically active. The document included the logos of many supporting organisations, including companies, government ministries, charities and societies such as Architecture for Humanity, and the International Society for Physical Activity and Health (ISPAH). What follows is an analysis of some of the themes within the document, which highlight how physical activity is framed in ways which are particularly useful for a company such as Nike.

A focus on leisure

As noted by Piggin (2015), the narrative of Designed To Move focuses mainly on leisure-time physical activity, despite occupational activity time having been identified as declining significantly in recent years. A number of associated graphs (Ng and Popkin, 2012) show declining activity rates in the USA, UK, Brazil, China and India. Following these charts is the comment,

> As paid work, domestic life and transportation require less physical effort, the primary opportunity for physical activity is in leisure and recreation. However, the data shows that time spent being physically active in leisure time doesn't come close to compensating for the overall drop in physical activity in other areas of life.
>
> (Nike *et al.*, 2012, p. 5)

And so leisure comes to dominate many of the examples in the document. A mere one page in DTM is devoted to 'Buildings/Workplaces' (p. 52). And despite the worker abuse which Nike's culture would no doubt be familiar with, the solution to occupation physical inactivity is presented particularly simplistically: sedentary behaviour in workplaces is explained away by the suggestion there is 'no reason' not to include physical activity:

Most people with desk jobs spend their days on emails, conference calls, or in webinars and meetings. These are usually sedentary activities – *but why*? There's really *no reason* most of these things can't be paired with some form of physical activity. *All that's needed are employers who encourage it.*

(p. 52, italics added)

As Piggin (2015) notes, the idea that all that is needed are employers who encourage physical activity "both frames managers as omnipotent agents and elides consideration of a host of institutional pressures, which often revolve around the innate corporate quest for productivity" (p. 21). Just one year before the Designed To Move document was published, another report suggested the ongoing exploitation of sport product workers (McGuinness, 2011; Shayon, 2011). The report read:

Nike, when confronted … admits the abuse from contractors, which includes slapping workers in the face and calling them pigs and dogs, but says (astoundingly) there's little they can do to stop it. The abuse claims are shocking. One worker at the Pou Chen Group factory in Sukabumi, 60 miles from Jakarta, alleges she was kicked by a supervisor for a mistake in cutting rubber for soles. "We're powerless," said the woman who spoke on condition of anonymity, fearing reprisal. "Our only choice is to stay and suffer, or speak out and be fired."

(Shayon, 2011)

According to the Associated Press report, "a group of female workers were forced to stand in the blazing sun for two hours as punishment for failing to make hundreds of pairs of shoes quickly enough". These conceptions of worker abuse by managers featured nowhere in the Designed To Move document. Instead, physical inactivity was framed as something which could be changed relatively easily.

The omission of old people from Nike's imagery

The Designed To Move document uses adult activity data in its "prelude to action" (p. 2). However, soon after this, the document frames young people as the focus: "Designed to Move calls for dramatic and urgent commitment to increase physical activity levels. Special emphasis must be placed on youth, especially kids under the age of 10" (p. 15). I argue that this targeting of young people is deliberate, and plays strongly into the marketing logic of Nike, a company which would seek to develop brand loyalty by consumers as early as possible.

Older adults are given a distinct lack of attention in the document. "Older adults" are mentioned only three times in total; the "elderly" twice, and each time only briefly (Piggin, 2015). Piggin notes that "older people" are also written about in a conservative manner, which reinforces problematic stereotypes of ageing. Early in DTM, the realm of sport, physical activity and physical play for older people is explained by the statement: "it could be jogging, swimming or ballroom dancing" (2015, p. viii). Piggin notes that the 'elderly' are aggregated within a list of "People With *Different* Levels of Ability/Capability" (2015, p. 37, italics added), which demonstrates normative assumptions about who should be active and who is classified as different. Older people are also marginalised by being visually absent. In no place in the entire document are any older people featured in the imagery. In comparison, 36 out of 40 images show children and young people being physically active or connoting physical activity. This omission of older adults is a technique familiar to Nike. In their promotion of *The Human Race – The Day the World Runs* in 2008 and 2009, Nike's advertising showed only young, lean and able-bodied people (Nike, 2009). It was clear that the 'world' to Nike consisted of a distinctly limited population.

This type of exclusion of older adults illustrates how Nike aims to shape readers' understandings in particular ways. While Nike claims that "We believe if you have a body, you're an athlete" (Nike *et al.*, 2012, p. 125), the near total omission of older people from the document suggests that some bodies are worthier of attention than others. Further, DTM is directed towards the "Changemakers – people, companies, institutions and governments [and] … nations who want to invest in unleashing the human potential of their citizens" (p. i), the scant attention to older adults suggests that they do not fit into this vision, perhaps because of their limited "human potential" (p. i). Phoenix and Sparkes (2008, p. 219) note that the expectations we have of life form culturally constructed pictures which "can enter our everyday language while simultaneously forming a base for the practical decisions of our life management and its societal organisation". The imagery and omission within the DTM document are important. They serve to frame the problem and possible solutions in certain ways, ways which are advantageous to the writers of the document.

Physical activity and brain power?

There were other ways that knowledge about physical activity was crafted by interest groups. Connecting physical activity and education is a powerful technique to elevate physical activity's importance. The Designed To Move document included an image with the associated text – "Fitness is associated with 40% higher test scores" (p. 14) with a reference to an article by James Grissom (2005). And indeed, the original research does evaluate the relationship between physical fitness and academic achievement. The "results indicate a consistent positive relationship between overall fitness and academic achievement" (p. 11).

But, Grissom also makes it clear that "results should be interpreted with caution. It cannot be inferred from these data that physical fitness causes academic achievement to improve" (p. 11) and

> a major axiom of social science research is that correlation is not cau-sality. It cannot be inferred from these data that physical fitness increased or improved academic achievement. There was no time or logical ordering that automatically led from one event to the other. It is just as logical to believe that mental capacity affects physical ability…. This study is seen as preliminary.
>
> (p. 24)

This is concerning because the title of Nike's image infers there is an extremely large causal relationship whereby fitness *leads to* higher test scores. The title of the graph refers to "compounding benefits" and "a prosperous cycle" from physical activity. Grissom's research did not claim this. In fact, he warned against concluding from this study that physical activity leads to higher test scores.

In the UK in 2014, a physical activity campaign was initiated called "Move1hour". (Move1hour did have a Facebook and twitter account but these are no longer live – a short-lived social movement indeed). However, the Designed To Move Facebook page re-asserted the "40% test score increase" claim to encourage physical activity. Nike would continue this claim until at recently as August 2015 (Nike, 2015).

Of course, dismantling one misleading argument about physical activity is not an attempt to question the positive outcomes of participation. However, it should make us wary of overly evangelical advocates. It is straight-forward to make a connection between this type of overreach by Nike and the rationale for doing so. Propagating this claim makes it easier for an organisation like Nike to gain the attention of young people in schools, along with a variety of Nike-adorned athletes. Saying children "can score 40% higher on tests" is a manipulation of the original research to the point where it is deceptive.

The Designed To Move 'movement' also found its way into the UK Government through the APCPA which published *Tackling Physical Inac-tivity: A Co-ordinated Approach* (2014). The APCPA was established in late 2013 as an 'All Party Parliamentary Group'; these are informal cross-party groups that have no official status within Parliament. They are run by and for Members of the Commons and Lords, though many involve individuals and organisations from outside Parliament in their administration and activities (UK Government, 2014). Thus it would be more appropriately described as a lobby or interest group. The APCPA was chaired by three Members of Parliament, one from each of the three largest political parties at the time, with another three Members of Parliament acting as Commissioners. The APCPA website stated it "was set up is in response to the overwhelming evidence in the *Designed to Move* report and the need for action to end the physical inactivity epidemic in the UK" (APCPA, 2013). Regarding low levels of population physical activity, the APCPA aimed to

> address this urgent issue and make direct, policy-based recommendations to tackle this crisis…. [a] novel approach is vital so that we can look for the first time at the whole, rather than the individual strands working in silo
>
> (APCPA, 2013)

This case study would show how the lobbying process for physical activity can manifest and unfold over a period of time. Numerous factors made this a compelling site of the policy process in action. The case involved many of the prominent organisations and stakeholders. The wide array of stakeholders also provided useful insight through both oral hearings and written submissions. Of the over 200 oral and written submissions, many were from representatives of larger groups such as the Associations of School and College Leaders, Birmingham City Council and the Federation of Sports and Play Associations. The APCPA would generate rich primary data about physical activity policy solutions, through in-person evidence sessions, media reporting and social media interaction. Various aspects of the APCPA were examined systematically, including the APCPA website, written evidence to the APCPA (by interested individuals and organisations, ranging from local residents, to academics, local councils and organisations involved with physical activity), and public evidence sessions and discussions (on education, health and sport). The final report named *Tackling Physical Inactivity: A Co-ordinated Approach* (APCPA, 2014b) was also critically assessed, along with publicity material from interest groups and policy communities such as news media statements, advertisements, organisational websites and social media sources.

As discussed in Chapter 3, the legitimacy of physical activity as a policy concern relies on associating it with other outcomes, as distinct from promoting activity simply as an end by itself. Activity is therefore linked with other domains, including, the economy, environment, education, health and social inclusion aims, among others. These domains were highly prioritised during the APCPA consultation and output phases. Aside from typical appeals to health and well-being, various other values and beliefs were apparent in the process. Ideas about nature and tradition were prominent. For example, the APCPA appealed to ideas about what is "natural" and stated that "the human body was *designed* to move" (2013, italics added), which is virtually identical to the main messages of the Designed To Move lobby document from Nike. These ideas also apparently informed the evidence givers to the APCPA. Evidence giver Paula Radcliffe implored the APCPA that a key message should be to "inspire what is naturally there in a child" and not to ignore children who were "*naturally* competitive" (Radcliffe, 2014, italics added). 'Tradition' also informed the physical activity lobby efforts. Evocations of tradition were present throughout the APCPA oral evidence sessions, with frequent reminiscing about what life used to be like. Epidemiological evidence is used to define people in the past as being more physically active than now (for more, see Piggin and Hart, 2017).

It was apparent there was intense interaction between the physical activity community in the organisation of the APCPA, to the extent that this was a combination of interest groups and policy communities. This *hybrid* form of organisation was consciously constructed to appear *official*. This was accomplished in various ways, including naming itself as a seemingly official 'Commission' (as opposed to the more usual term 'Group'), taking place in the Palace of Westminster (on the premises of the UK Government), being organised by six Members of Parliament and a 'non-party political crossbench peer', and emphasising *rationality* through evidence gathering. Although these factors added to the APCPA's perceived authority, the APCPA was actually part of an 'all party group' (APG). APGs do not have official status within Parliament (UK Government, 2014). Rather, APGs would more appropriately be termed as interest or pressure groups (BBC, 2011). The APCPA sat under the auspices of the 'APG Sport' and according to the APCPA website 'The Co-Chairs and Commissioners are supported in this work by the *Designed to Move* Champions...' (APCPA, 2013). This point is important, since it became clear that some of the groups giving 'evidence' to the APCPA were also already supporting it. For example, Nike, the lead author of the aforementioned Designed To Move, had a spokesperson give evidence, who echoed the sentiments of the Designed To Move document.

Throughout the lobbying process, some solutions gather strength and legitimacy, while others weaken and disappear from the discourse. The APCPA, Public Health England and UKActive chose and framed which ideas to present as solutions. To illustrate, the potential solutions offered to the APCPA by oral evidence givers included a vast array of ideas such as

"Make young people feel part of a family", "Street closure (to cars) is important for physical activity", "Use sportsmen and women for inspiration", "Emphasise physical literacy", "Don't mention sport at all in physical activity promotion" (APCPA, 2014a). These examples from the oral evidence sessions from a range of evidence givers illustrate the diversity of possible policy actions, which ranged from novel ideas of the speaker to best practice examples taken from other communities or countries. It was apparent the dominant concern of the APCPA was children and young people. This was also apparent in the final report of the APCPA, which featured only photographs of children being active (mimicking the original Designed To Move document). This was commented on by one physical activity academic: "All-party report on physical activity: 12 photos, all on children and 8 on sport. Adults, non-sport PA not important? #activity-commission" (Biddle, 2014). Since a significant majority of the discussions were given to children and young people, there was little (and at times no) emphasis from various oral evidence givers to discuss the concerns of employees and workplaces (for example).

The emphasis on young people in both the APCPA's final report and the subsequent activity promotion campaign 'Move1Hour' (Move1Hour, 2014a) which was endorsed on the APCPA website, demonstrate that while different groups are acknowledged in the APCPA report, the dominant ideas largely echo the Designed To Move lobby document from 2012 (Nike *et al.*, 2012). Specifically, a few pages in both Designed To Move and the APCPA report show major similarities, to the extent that some phrases are virtually identical. The APCPA report used Nike's 'copyright' Human Capital Model, and the style, tone and solutions offered in the APCPA report are similar to Designed To Move. In one instance, the similarity is so great that an advertisement used in the Designed To Move campaign in 2012 was rebranded with the Move-1Hour logo in 2014 (Move1Hour, 2014b). The overwhelming focus throughout the Move1Hour campaign was on young people, also echoing the Designed To Move document. Given that many of the Designed To Move Champions were supporting the APCPA as well as providing evidence to it, it is perhaps not surprising that many of the ideas in Designed To Move are duplicated in the final APCPA report. However, it does highlight the ability of interest groups or organisations to frame the debate about the solutions to population physical inactivity in particular ways. These close links to the Move1Hour campaign indicates hybridity of the APCPA as at once a pseudo-official evidence-gathering group and a physical activity promoter with specific target groups in mind. It might also raise questions about how 'revolutionary' and effective such an approach might be.

A short-lived media campaign followed the APCPA report. One of the most memorable and startling advertisements on billboards and newspapers branded with 'Move1' was an image of a skull merged with a chair and the accompanying lines that "Sitting is the new enemy" and "Sitting is the new smoking". That this campaign demonised a perfectly reasonable and useful human activity is demonstrative of some of the problematic rationalities that informed the larger Designed To Move campaign.

Conclusion

Ostensibly, a company such as Nike, the products of which support physical activity, would be an ideal corporate partner. However, any good that was done through Nike's campaigning must also be set against,

- an admitted history of connections with factory worker abuse which was not factored into Nike's conception of workplaces in Designed To Move,
- conflation of correlation and causality in scientific research,
- the publishing in a scientific journal of highly problematic ideas about how financial capital is attained,
- an obvious targeting of children's physical activity (and exclusion of older adults) through their lobbying, and
- the demonisation of sitting.

Could these issues be explained away as misunderstandings or over-analysis by someone not involved in the 'movement'? It was apparent over time that other voices also saw problematic aspects of such a corporate relationship. At an event launching a Special Issue of *The Lancet* on Physical Activity in 2016, a contributing author and panellist was extremely disappointed by the attempts of physical activity advocates to cooperate with Nike and the Designed To Move initiative, saying it did not work at all. His conclusion was that "their interests are not our interests" (Speaker, 2016). Similarly, an advocate working in various health promotion agencies in Europe was troubled by the absence of older adults from serious consideration (such as their relative absence from the Designed To Move report). He believed that Nike's attitude towards older adults was problematic – and perceived that older adults were excluded because they "were not good for [Nike's] image" (Laventure, 2017).

The impact of corporate interests on physical activity must be seriously scrutinised. The following chapter continues this theme.

Notes

1 This chapter is informed by analysis presented by Piggin (2015), and research by Joe Piggin and Louise Hart (2017) published in Leisure Studies.

References

All Party Commission on Physical Activity [APCPA] (2013). Terms of reference. Retrieved from http://activitycommission.com/about/terms-of-reference/

All Party Commission on Physical Activity [APCPA] (2014a, 15 January). Health oral evidence session for the All Party Commission on Physical Activity. London, UK: Palace of Westminster.

All Party Commission on Physical Activity [APCPA] (2014b). *Tackling Physical Inactivity: A Co-ordinated Approach.* England, UK: APCPA.

Bailey, R., Hillman, C., Arent, S. and Petipas, A. (2013). Physical activity: An underestimated investment in human capital. *Journal of Physical Activity and Health, 10,* 289–308.

BBC (2011). All-party parliamentary groups. Retrieved from news.bbc.co.uk/democracylive/hi/guides/newsid_81000/81876.stm

Biddle, S. (2014, 8 April). Twitter comment. Retrieved from www.twitter.com

Grissom, J.B. (2005). Physical fitness and academic achievement. *Journal of Exercise Physiology Online, 8,* 11–25.

Laventure, B. (2017, 5 April). *'Everybody's Interest, Nobody's Responsibility': Physical Activity Policy through the Lifecourse Seminar.* Seminar at Loughborough University, UK.

McGuinness, R. (2011). Nike staff in Indonesia subjected to 'serious' physical and verbal abuse. Retrieved from http://metro.co.uk/2011/07/13/nike-staff-in-indonesia-subjected-to-serious-physical-and-verbal-abuse-76348/

Move1Hour (2014a). Move1Hour Physical Activity Campaign. Retrieved from https://twitter.com/move1hour

Move1Hour (2014b). 5 Extra Years: Video advertisement. Retrieved from www.youtube.com/user/Move1Hour/videos

Nike (2005). Nike Fy04 Corporate Responsibility Report. Retrieved from http://nikeinc.com/system/assets/1836/Nike_FY04_CR_report_original.pdf

Nike (2009). The Human Race: The day the world runs. Nike advertising campaign.

Nike *et al.* (2012). Designed To Move: A physical activity action agenda. Retrieved from www.designedtomove.org/

Nike (2015). Kids Run the World: Nike partners with marathon kids. Retrieved from https://news.nike.com/news/kids-run-the-world-nike-partners-with-marathon-kids

Ng, S.W. and Popkin, B.M. (2012). Time use and physical activity: A shift away from movement across the globe. *Obesity Reviews, 13*(8), 659–680.

Phoenix, C. and Sparkes, A.C. (2008). Athletic bodies and aging in context: The narrative construction of experienced and anticipated selves in time. *Journal of Aging Studies, 22*(3), 211–221.

Piggin, J. (2015). Designed to move? Physical activity lobbying and the politics of productivity. *Health Education Journal, 74*(1), 16–27.

Piggin, J., and Hart, L. (2017). Physical activity advocacy in the UK: A multiple streams analysis of a hybrid policy issue. *Leisure Studies, 36*(5), 708–720.

Radcliffe, P. (2014, 29 January). Education oral evidence session for the All Party Commission on Physical Activity. London, UK: Palace of Westminster.

Shayon, S. (2011). Nike better world? Not for Converse factory workers in Indonesia. Retrieved from www.brandchannel.com/home/post/2011/07/13/nike-just-not-doing-it-right.aspx

Speaker (2016, July). *Launch of The Lancet Physical Activity Series 2.* London School of Hygiene and Tropical Medicine, London, UK.

UK Government (2014). All party groups. Retrieved from www.parliament.uk/about/mps-andlords/members/apg/

8 Physical activity and the politics of risk

Rugby union is a popular sport in UK schools and, like countries such as Australia, New Zealand and South Africa, is often claimed to be the national sport. However, it has recently come under scrutiny for being too dangerous for children to play (Omalu, 2016; SCIC, 2016). England Rugby, the English national governing body has been reluctant to remove the tackle element from the sport in schools. Instead, England Rugby emphasises the positive aspects that come from the sport: "Using rugby union as a vehicle for developing young people's personal and social skills alongside their rugby skills can have a dramatic impact on all aspects of their lives and has real whole school impact" (England Rugby, 2017). The debate over the place of rugby continues. For this chapter, I take the governing interests of the sport of rugby, such as England Rugby and World Rugby, to be 'corporate interests'. That is, organisations like these have concerns beyond facilitating young people to be physically active. They are large-scale organisations with sizable work forces, which receive significant sums of money from a variety of sources, including private corporate sponsors, and income from customers and media companies.

Risk of injury in sport

With this context in mind, it is necessary to begin this chapter with a cliché – 'everything in life has risk'. From a policy perspective though, it is also necessary to mention something about how risk is calculated. Beck (1992) describes the logic that first brought risk management into the realm of *policy making*:

> Consequences that at first affect only the individual become "risks", systematically caused, statistically describable and in that sense "predictable" types of events which can therefore also be subjected to

supra-individual and political rules of recognition, compensation and avoidance.

(p. 99)

Many collision sports have historically promoted cultures that tolerate pain and injury as essential, even glorified aspects of the sport. Recent research reveals that non-elite rugby players in Ireland often display an irreverent attitude towards concussion which encourages risky behaviours and underplays, ignores or denies the significance of concussion (Liston *et al.*, 2016). Paralleling this, there have been growing concerns about the potential long-lasting effects of injuries; governing bodies have proclaimed they are trying to decrease injury rates, such as World Rugby's CEO saying the organisation is "committed to highlighting and improving player welfare through education and promotion of correct preparation, playing techniques and prevention strategies" (see Raftery, 2016).

A second (and final) cliché is offered here. A common defence of participation in collision sports is that the participants are 'aware of the risks involved' and therefore consent to participate. This chapter problematises this claim with three case studies of collisions sport, two from the sport of rugby union and one from American football.

Collating and disseminating accurate injury and risk information is of increasing importance for sports organisations around the world. A widely accepted assertion in the sports medicine community is that "the accuracy and consistency in calculation and reporting of injury incidence is crucial" (Fortington *et al.*, 2017). This is important for various reasons, from identification of injuries that could be targeted for prevention, to monitoring interventions (van Mechelen *et al.*, 1992; Finch *et al.*, 2001; Arnason *et al.*, 2004; Finch, 2006; Shrier *et al.*, 2009; Fortington *et al.*, 2017). Fuller and Drawer (2004) discussed risk management, and their conclusion is worth repeating here in totality:

> Although participants may appear to accept the levels of risk associated with a sport, this is often a result of ignorance of the actual levels of risk involved. This is an important issue because it is clearly difficult for a participant to accept risks about which they have little or no knowledge. In these cases, *governing bodies have a major responsibility for identifying and managing the risks associated with the sport and then communicating the information to participants.* Current levels of risk in many sports are clearly too high and there have been examples of litigation as a result of severe and fatal injuries.

(pp. 354–355, italics added)

As Fuller and Drawer allude to, accuracy of injury management is also increasingly important in a legal sense. The marketing and promotion that sports governing bodies engage in seems partially targeted for consumption by youth, adolescents and recreational athletes with the aim of increasing or reinforcing participation. Therefore, injury risk reporting must meet marketing standards and be accurate. Advertising standards in many countries require claims made by marketers about programmes and services to be honest, truthful and accurate (Advertising Standards Authority for Ireland, 2016; Federal Trade Commission, 2016). The accuracy of injury reporting is a pertinent issue for governing bodies of collision sports in the North America and Europe, which have faced increased scrutiny from lobbyists about risk and injury rates in their sports (Omalu, 2016; Tucker *et al.*, 2016). Of course, governmental departments, such as the Ministry of Education and the Ministry of Health are implicated in this too, since there is an expectation of a duty of care at schools.

Concerns about perceived high levels of risk might come from participants, potential participants, parents and guardians of children who participate, spectators who might be turned away by a perception of high-risk activity, facilitators such as teachers who might offer collision sports to students and insurance companies which are involved in making risk assessments for claims purposes. Because of the debates about risk, governing bodies have been involved in a variety of education, public relations and marketing activities to allay fears about the (relative) risk involved in participation in their respective sports.

To gain insight into how sports governing bodies frame risk, this chapter draws on case studies of contesting erroneous claims about risk presented by national governing bodies.

Rugby tackling in schools?

What follows is my account of my involvement in public debate over the place of tackling in schools in the UK between 2015 and 2017. The debate highlighted different perspectives on the duty of care for children in schools, notions of un/acceptable risk, questions about the supposed expertise of those calling for tackling to be removed from school sport and PE, and the importance of rugby as a school sport and core aspect of identity for many people in the UK. My involvement in the issue has thus far been small compared to other protagonists, and so I do not wish to suggest I was a central figure in the debate. However, as with any type of advocacy, the amount and intensity of involvement can alter over time.

In late 2015, I co-signed (with around 70 other academics) an open letter to various medical officers and education leaders. The letter petitioned for the removal of tackling from rugby in school sport because of the associated injury risk. The publication of the letter on 1 March 2016 generated a very large media response (albeit short-lived because of the news media cycle), with talk shows and news items devoting much attention to it. It was an incendiary topic on social media, ranging from agreement to disagreement to vitriol and ridicule of the signatories.

While I could appreciate many of the narratives which emerged in defence of school rugby tackling (from confidence building to skill development), one idea sat uneasily with me. The idea, paraphrased, was that 'as long as people know and accept the risk, tackling is acceptable'. As a sport scholar having participated in a variety of sports over the course of my life, I had little comprehension (beyond intuition) of what the relative injury risks of participation *actually* were, and so it was at least possible that many others, including parents, teachers and participants, would not know about the risk of participation either. The plot thickened when I simply perused claims made by two of the most influential rugby organisations in the world, World Rugby and England Rugby. These claims included:

> Compared with other sports and activities, rugby has a relatively low injury rate despite being known for its physicality,
>
> (World Rugby, 2016a)

and

> There is no evidence to show that rugby poses a specifically greater risk than other sports.
>
> (England Rugby, 2016b)

The claims these organisations made about injury risk appeared to be incredible, or more appropriately, *not credible*. Subsequently, I entered into correspondence with various co-signatories, regarding the need for the removal of false injury risk claims that both organisations presented, and the need for the publication of accurate data. Both personal communication via email and an editorial in the *British Journal of Sport Medicine* (*BJSM*) advised World Rugby to remove *and correct* their erroneous and misleading claims about injury risk (see Piggin and Pollock, 2016). Similarly, via email and a post on Idrotts Forum, a Nordic Sport Science Forum, I and Prof Alan Bairner advised England Rugby to remove their erroneous claims, publicly acknowledge their mistake *and publish correct information* (see Piggin and Bairner, 2017).

In both cases the organisations followed our advice to remove the erroneous claims from their websites. Our advice to both World Rugby and England Rugby was simply to use correctly the data they had erroneously used, and to publicise this to their members. However, it appeared that neither organisation followed our advice about publicly acknowledging their dissemination of misleading information or clarifying what the specific risk in rugby was, although the CEO of World Rugby did respond in the 'pay-walled' *BJSM.*

Another critique was levied against the evidence that the Chief Medical Officers (CMO) of the United Kingdom used to justify not promoting change to the school game. In response to the original letter, the CMOs of the UK consulted, gathered evidence and finally decided to continue to support the status quo of tackling in school rugby (UK CMOs, 2016). The CMOs concluded that "the evidence does not support the conclusions and recommendations laid out in [the] open letter". The CMOs justified their decision by relying on a report from the UK Physical Activity Expert Group (PAEG, 2016, see the UK CMO's response) and a review article by Dr Ross Tucker and colleagues in the *BJSM.* However, as pointed out by Piggin and Bairner (2018) there were several problems with relying on these specific sources of evidence, as discussed in the following paragraphs.

Questions about the prevalence of concussion

In responding to an assertion that 'concussion is a common injury' in rugby the PAEG stated: "It seems that before the sustained programme of education and awareness in rugby concussions were under reported, and it may be now that true concussion is over-reported, making it currently difficult to ascertain where the true incidence lies." However, Piggin and Bairner suggested that the PAEG should focus their attention on recent research published about attitudes towards concussion in community rugby (see Liston *et al.*, 2016) which showed "non-elite players tend to display an irreverent attitude towards concussion which encourages risky behaviours and underplays, ignores or denies the significance of concussion". Further, another recent study on community rugby concluded that "concussion was the most common head injury diagnosis, although it is likely that this injury was underreported" (Roberts *et al.*, 2017). Relatedly, Hume and colleagues (2016) reported that New Zealand community and elite *former rugby union players reported a substantially higher number of concussions* (76.8 per cent and 84.5 per cent respectively) than non-contact-sport players (23.1 per cent). What this recent research shows is that there is evidence of serious issues with how concussion is understood and at times underestimated, and so therefore a cautious approach would be prudent.

Rugby as compulsory for some children

The original letter stated that "many secondary schools in the United Kingdom deliver contact rugby as a compulsory part of the physical education curriculum from age eleven". In response the PAEG wrote that "rugby is not stated as a compulsory part of the PE offer". However, even though it is not stated as compulsory in the PE curriculum, it is still plausible that schools might make it compulsory to participate. As such, Piggin and Bairner noted that the PAEG appeared to elevate policy rhetoric above the practical reality of many school settings. A survey of rugby-playing schools in 2015 showed that rugby was "compulsory in 77% of responding schools" (Nyiri, 2015).

Total number of injuries or rates relative to participation

Perhaps one of the most significant problems with the PAEG evidence which was used by the UK CMOs was the problematic use of participation statistics (a problem that had been seen with both the World Rugby and England Rugby articulations as well). The PAEG claimed that "One of the few examples of injury surveillance, from Oxfordshire, showed that rugby was not the largest contributor to injuries in the under 20s who play sport" [PAEG, 2016, underline in original]. The PAEG compared the statistics for 10- to 14-year-old males, with football "responsible for 36% of injuries [and] rugby union 18%". However, Piggin and Bairner (2018) showed that these percentages compared the *total* number of injuries rather than the injuries *relative* to the number of participants. Of course, injuries relative to participation rates would be more valuable to know than the raw numbers, especially when various sports differ wildly in participation rates. It could be noted that Sport England data show that nearly ten times more people in England play football than rugby union. In 2014, 1.8 million people participated in football, whereas 191,900 participated in rugby union (Sport England, 2016). Therefore, of course the *relative risk of injury* needs to inform policy. Again, a variety of evidence would show that rugby can be far more dangerous than other sports. Nicholl *et al.* (1995) found that "*the risk of a substantive injury in rugby was three times that in soccer*". Fuller (2008) wrote that "Rugby union is a full contact sport with *a relatively high overall risk of injury*". What all of this shows again is a distinctly confined and constrained consideration of a range of information used to make policy decisions.

Does tackling affect physical activity in schools?

The PAEG stated that "*not allowing children to play or be active will be detrimental to their emotional, social, mental and physical health*". However, Piggin and Bairner, (2017) call this a straw person fallacy because the logic does not hold true under scrutiny. School children could theoretically partake in several physical activities, and it is potentially the case that there are opportunity costs in having compulsory rugby lessons. There are many ways of children being physical active. Of course, removing tackling in rugby does not prevent physical activity.

What is understood by 'duty of care'?

Piggin and Bairner note another contradiction which informs the policy thinking about the safety of children in schools. The PAEG (2016) would contribute two contradictory claims. At one point they wrote "*Clearly schools, teachers and coaches have a duty of care for children at all times ...*". However, at another point, in reference to the United Nations Convention on the Rights of the Child whereby governments have a duty to protect children from risks of injury, the PAEG stated: "*We feel this assertion lies outside of the scope of the Expert Committee.*" It is difficult to reconcile this contradiction. It also leads onto questions about how safe children should be at school.

It was also possible to critically analyse the single academic article cited by the UK CMOs as well, in coming to their decision. Of course, all scientific research has limitations, and it is important to acknowledge these before accepting the information. This article was published in the *BJSM* and entitled "Injury risk and a tackle ban in youth Rugby Union: reviewing the evidence and searching for targeted, effective interventions. A critical review" (Tucker *et al.*, 2016). This article was endorsed by the UK CMOs, despite the fact that the title of the article focused on 'youth rugby', not school rugby as discussed in the original open letter. In any case, all research has limitations which should encourage policy makers to consider such evidence critically.

First, Tucker *et al.* (2016) cite Finch (2006) and claim that "*effective interventions must, by definition, be realistic and obtain the support of the major stakeholders [including sporting bodies] within the specific target population*". While Finch (2006) did indeed write this, obtaining support is certainly *not* always necessary. For example, there is no need to obtain support from soft drink companies to remove their products from hospitals, or from cigarette manufacturers when imposing extra taxes on their products. Similarly, while England Rugby and World Rugby are major stakeholders in school rugby provision, there is no need to obtain their support for an intervention in formal school settings. Indeed, effective interventions might often be those which elevate specific risk reduction measures above corporate stakeholder interests.

Second, Tucker *et al.* (2016) claim *"the risk of participation in Rugby Union, while warranting focus and continued efforts for primary injury prevention, does not stand out beyond that of other popular sports"*. This claim appears extremely contentious. As mentioned earlier, there is indeed research that shows rugby has higher injury rates than other sports.

Third, Tucker *et al.* (2016) acknowledge that *"around 15 years of age appears to be when the incidence of injury in contact and collision sports increases in comparison to non-contact sports"*. Not only does this remark seem to contradict the previous comment from the authors of the article, but further, 15 to 17 year olds are of typical school age and so were clearly implicated in the open letter's proposed intervention of removing the tackle from school settings. A 2014 Australian report noted that for 15 to 17 year olds, rugby is a sport with a high participation-based hospitalisation rate compared to many others, especially so compared with other sports played at schools (Kreisfeld *et al.*, 2014). By including 15 to 17 year olds playing rugby at school in their analysis, Tucker *et al.* would have greatly contextualised the issue.

By not doing so, they potentially contribute (probably unwittingly) to a skewed perception of injury risk in school rugby by the CMOs.

Fourth, the fact that Tucker *et al.* (2016) misdescribed injury rates in a study by Pringle *et al.* (claiming that netball was most injurious) further highlights the need for clarification in the article (see Pringle *et al.*, 1998). That the Tucker *et al.* article was the only research paper cited directly by the CMOs as supporting the conclusions of the PAEG seems problematic.

Fifth, on numerous occasions Tucker *et al.* (2016) overlook the fact that the original letter focused on *school* rugby. At the end of their article Tucker *et al.* claim that *"the proposal to remove all contact from youth rugby should not be supported by Rugby Union governing bodies"*. Given that the original letter focused specifically on the *educational setting of school sport*, this is another instance where the intention of the original letter might well be skewed, and possibly contribute to confusion by anyone who used the article to justify policy decisions.

Sixth, it seems the CMOs used contradictory claims to reach their decision about continuing to endorse tackling in school rugby. There appears to be a contradiction between advice offered by Tucker *et al.* (2016) and conclusions drawn by the PAEG regarding where the CMOs sought their advice about injury surveillance. Tucker *et al.* (2016) claimed that "*The review focuses primarily on the paucity of research data with which to guide clinical practice.... Clinical practitioners, including those involved in the sport of Rugby Union, must address the need for well-controlled injury surveillance data.*" However, the PAEG stated that the allegation (by the letter writers) that there is insufficient injury data "*appears unfair as recent Home Nation rugby football unions initiatives are focusing on prevention and monitoring*". This contradiction is difficult to reconcile and should lead to questions about the state of injury surveillance. Is there, or is there not, enough? If there are contradictory statements being used about the level and quality of evidence, then how can sound policy decisions be made?

Beyond these, one final concern is worth noting with how the Tucker *et al.* article has been used by the UK CMOs. The 'Competing Interests' section of the Tucker *et al.* article includes the statement that two of the three authors "*are salaried employees at World Rugby Ltd, the governing body for the sport of Rugby Union globally*". It seems somewhat troubling that the *only* research cited by the CMOs was written by two paid employees of World Rugby, an organisation with a pecuniary interest in increasing participation in schools. The infusion of corporate interests into policy making of sports with high injury rates is surely something that policy makers (such as the UK CMOs) should not ignore.

Understanding risk trivialisation

It was after these events that the germination of a framework to explain why these governing bodies, who very often profess to have 'player welfare' as a priority, would not swiftly make risk information *easily publicly accessible* to their stakeholders, including teachers, parents and players who would use such information to make decisions about participation. While acknowledging that there are and probably will continue to be vociferous debates about what the 'real' risk of participation is I offer the following Risk Trivialisation Framework as a contribution to understanding the corporate dynamics involved in rugby union.

Theory building: risk trivialisation framework

By reflecting on the two earlier interactions with sports governing bodies (World Rugby and England Rugby), and another from American football in the USA, I argue there are serious shortcomings about the current way in which risk and injury information is communicated to the public about various sports. Specifically, the analysis suggests that a confluence of circumstances and behaviours have led to claims by sports governing bodies being crafted in such a way that they trivialise the risk involved in sport participation.

Risk trivialisation by sports governing bodies is concerning for two reasons. First, the countries in which many governing bodies are based have legal obligations regarding the truthfulness of marketing claims. Second, it is imperative for the integrity of health professionals involved in sport as well as transparency of the organisations themselves that injury and risk claims are not subjected to distortion and understatement. By conceiving governing sports organisations as corporate 'bodies', this analysis argues these bodies are capable of distortionary behaviour. This behaviour is presented here as Risk Trivialisation (RT):

> Defective corporate processes and practices leading to inaccurate and misleading injury risk claims.

The elements of RTF will be taken to include:

> Risk: Quantifiable population-based data regarding probability of injury occurring.
> Trivialisation: The act of suppressing or underplaying the extent of a problem such that it appears less severe than it might be.
> Framework: A conceptual model for understanding possible process of risk presentations.

By examining the behaviour of corporate bodies (rather than individuals within them) this analysis proposes antecedents and contributing factors, symptoms and treatment of RT. Three case studies are offered to illustrate RT in action. USA Football, World Rugby and England Rugby.

Antecedents and causes of RT

(a) Bodies with expansionist visions. A sports body's desire for growth is a key ingredient in RT. The logic of expansion, territorially, in spectator numbers and in participant numbers can be seen in the strategic plans of various sports bodies. Carl D. Peterson, the chairman of USA Football stated in 2014 that the organisation's goal is "to grow our game nationally and internationally … and our brightest days are yet to come" (USA Football, 2014). Since 2004 World Rugby had "a blueprint for growth that would enable the sport to be truly global and reach out to new audiences and participants around the world" (World Rugby, 2014). Under the heading 'Grow', the current strategic plan aims to "Increase global parti-cipation" (World Rugby, 2016a). Expansionist visions are also present in England Rugby, which currently promotes "All Schools" (England Rugby, 2016a). According to its strategy,

> Rugby union is a game for All Schools – everyone can play it and every school can teach it. CBRE All Schools has been developed by the RFU to increase the amount of rugby in schools, and to encourage new players to join local clubs.
>
> (England Rugby, 2012)

These various strategic plans and statements indicate these sports bodies' desires to expand geographically, in participation numbers and audience numbers.

(b) Bodies with significant pecuniary interests. Whether governing bodies have explicit profit motives or describe themselves as non-profits, large income streams enable sports to establish systems which facilitate the expansionist visions noted above through coaching, education and marketing programmes. More specifically, income generation affords gov-erning bodies the ability and resources to compile and transform informa-tion into targeted marketing strategies. Such organisations also have close links with companies with explicit profit motives such as sportswear com-panies and media companies. For instance, USA Football notes that in 2014 "effective managing of costs have increased revenues from $7.7 million to $22.0 [million], enabling us to reinvest in new standard-setting programs and resources" (USA Football, 2014). The strategic plan of World Rugby includes the aim to "Maximise commercial values and increase the financial sustainability of international rugby" (World Rugby, 2016c). England Rugby's strategy claims to have "£1/3 billion invested in rugby over the five-year period" (England Rugby, 2012). Given such signi-ficant financial incentives, there is a direct interest in promoting sports as positive, healthy and 'safe' (England Rugby, 2016b).

(c) Sports with a relatively high amount of collision and injury. It is readily apparent that both American football and rugby are sports which involve collisions as a fundamental component of the game. It is this col-liding that at once appeals to participants and spectators while leading others to question the effects of collisions, both short term and long term. Of course, attitudes towards sport collisions are informed by a variety of factors such as values, expertise and lived experience. In terms of how atti-tudes towards risk of injury are framed, sports governing bodies echo each other. USA Football claims that the "health and well-being of every young athlete is USA Football's No. 1 priority" (USA Football, 2014). England

Rugby states it is "working hard to ensure that safety and welfare remains the highest priority across the game" (England Rugby, 2016b) and World Rugby's Player Welfare slogan is "Putting Players First" (World Rugby, 2016b). However, these sports have faced criticism from lobby groups (including scientists, parents and health promoters) and this has contributed to a subsequent urge to quantify risk involved in sports which have in the past established social capital for being perceived as brutal, gladiatorial and violent (Dunning, 2008). These contests over the values and ideas of various collision sports (as violent or safe) contribute to RT.

(d) The employment of marketers to translate scientific data into comprehensible infographics, slogans and claims for consumers and participants. Many collision sports emphasise 'education' as a way of decreasing injury. The tools and techniques range from coaching courses, to online instructional videos and medical training for officials. In order to allay the fears of decision makers (such as parents and school boards) about the safety of a sport, governing bodies produce and promote statistics which are easily digestible for the intended audience. It is the intermediary who is often tasked with translating research data into easy-to-comprehend information for decision makers and consumers, and it is through this process that dis-ordered information about injury rates can emerge. RT observably manifests through claims in marketing and promotional material which, unless and until they are critiqued and retracted, remain in the public domain. Each case is considered in detail here, in order to for the reader to observe how RT manifests.

USA Football: Funded and promoted by the NFL, 'Heads Up Football' is a programme designed to increase safety when playing American football, in part through participants learning 'proper' tackling technique (USA Football, 2016). In its 2014 Annual Report, USA Football claimed that a

> study revealed that youth football players in leagues that participate in USA Football's Heads Up Football program have a 76 percent reduction in injuries compared to those in leagues that do not take part in the program … [and] Heads Up Football leagues also saw a reduction in concussions during both practices (34 percent) and games (29 percent).
>
> (USA Football, 2014)

However, an analysis in the *New York Times* found that "That study, published in July 2015, showed no such thing" (Schwarz, 2016). A USA Football spokesperson acknowledged they "had erred in not conducting a more thorough review" and promised to remove the erroneous print and online material, and that partners and constituents would be notified of the errors (Schwarz, 2016).

World Rugby: In 2015, World Rugby published an infographic claiming that "Compared with other sports and activities, rugby has a relatively low injury rate despite being known for its physicality" (Piggin and Pollock, 2016). A chart which purported to show sport-related hospital admissions in Australia implied that rugby accounted for just 5 per cent compared with cycling (25 per cent), equestrian (23 per cent) motorsport (23 per cent). However, an editorial in the *BJSM* showed that World Rugby's claims were inaccurate and seriously misleading. Contrary to World Rugby's claims of a relatively *low* injury rate, the source document claimed that rugby has a "*high* participation-based [hospitalisation] rate" (Kreisfeld *et al.*, 2014). Subsequently, Brett Gosper, the CEO of World Rugby acknowledged and apologised for the errors caused by misinterpretation by the infographic creators (Raftery, 2016). However, no apparent public statement was made to correct the misleading claims, beyond short statement in a pay-walled academic journal.

England Rugby: England Rugby's 'Rugby Safe' booklet was first published in 2015 and framed rugby injuries in various ways (England Rugby, 2016b). Several of the comments in this booklet regarding risk were problematic because they did not appear to meet standards of accuracy. Under the heading 'Rugby as a safe sport' was the claim that "One of the reasons players love rugby is that it is a physical sport. That does not mean that we accept that injuries are inevitable" (England Rugby, 2016b). This was a concerning statement, considering that the vast array of scientific articles on rugby injury rates demonstrably show that injuries, at a team level, *are* inevitable. Of course, it is possible that an individual might complete a match or a season uninjured, but this analysis suggests that a governing body should accept the inevitability of injuries at a team level. Indeed, governing bodies recognising that injuries within sport *are* inevitable might lead to more realistic expectations for outcomes following injury prevention strategies, managing participants' expectations, and managing the risks themselves.

However, even more concerning was another quote on the same page attributed to C.W. Fuller from the Centre for Sports Medicine, University of Nottingham. The quote stated that "There is no evidence to show that rugby poses a specifically greater risk than other sports" (England Rugby, 2016b). This claim was in total contradiction to a range of research and reports into injury rates between sports. The claim ignored a range of evidence regarding the apparent higher risk of injury in rugby. For example, in 2008 C.W. Fuller wrote that "Rugby union is a full contact sport with a relatively high overall risk of injury…" (Fuller, 2008). Also, in 2005

Brooks *et al.* published a study which claimed that "Rugby union is one of the most popular professional team sports in the world, but it also has one of the highest reported incidences of injury, irrespective of the injury definition used" (Brooks *et al.*, 2005). While not dealing with all age groups, this evidence is contrary to the Fuller quote in the England Rugby document. This claim of a relatively *high* overall injury risk is also supported by the Australian hospitalisation data which suggests a relatively high injury rate in rugby (Kreisfeld *et al.*, 2014). New Zealand data also shows a relatively high injury rate in rugby (ACC, 2016). On the following page of the 'Rugby Safe' booklet, catastrophic injury comparisons were presented, yet this data did not provide comparative data with other sports. The England Rugby 'Rugby Safe' document was not presented with due diligence about available statistics regarding injury rates. It was eventually removed, following a post I and Professor Alan Bairner made on 'Idrotts Forum' and a follow up email to the medical and marketing staff at England Rugby. Subsequently, while a spokesperson from England Rugby did send an email to state that the erroneous document had been removed from circulation and that there would be "an updated Rugby Safe booklet next season using the latest research and findings", the organisation did not publicly acknowledge the misleading claims, which had been promoted for nearly two years.

A note on intent, antecedents and the 'truth' of risk data

The proposed RT framework does not make a claim about whether misleading and inaccurate risk claims are produced intentionally. Further, it does not allege a greenwashing conspiracy on the part of national governing bodies. Clearly, there are significant concerted efforts to minimise risk of injury through education programmes, equipment advances and rule changes. However, the framework assumes that *at least*, inaccurate representations result from a lack of due diligence by a range of people involved in the production of injury risk claims. These may range from the researchers that collect data and the sport promoters who create the marketing material, to fact checkers who allow inaccurate data to be reported. No matter how many individuals are deficient in due diligence, this framework does not propose to account for individuals who knowingly set out to deceive. That is, the concept suggests those involved in promoting the sport will 'look for the good' in injury data, and not necessarily treat this information critically. Therefore, while the misrepresentation may not have been intentional, the desire to downplay risk was a strong motivating factor in producing injury risk data in the first place. This does not absolve individuals from responsibility as a result of a lack of due diligence, however.

The relative influence of any of these various antecedents will certainly vary on a case by case basis. However, the case studies provided here suggest that the existence of all these elements makes it more likely for RT to occur.

Further, this theorisation of risk assumes a level of agreement by all involved regarding the accuracy of the *original* statistics. Therefore, we leave arguments about the closeness of data to some positivist 'truth' regarding the risk of injury, the rigour of research designs, and the absence of bias to future analyses.

Minimising risk trivialisation

A range of policy actions are proposed to decrease the prevalence, severity and duration of erroneous and false injury claims being made by sports governing bodies.

(a) Using independent experts to review risk and injury claims that are made by sports bodies: These independent experts will review claims made about injury rates in each sport before they are published. This reiterates a recent proposal for participatory safety policy design in sports governing bodies (Dahlström *et al.*, 2015).

(b) Including links to source data: It should become a standardised practice to include links to, and references for all claims made about injuries in sport. This will ensure that spokespeople can refer to the original source and that claims can be checked for veracity. Allowing readers (parents, participants and researchers alike) to examine the original data used to check the veracity of claims will ensure more transparency in the injury reporting process.

(c) Refraining from over-stylising injury data: It appears that in some of the cases examined here, errors can occur through the process of translating data from the original source into easy-to-comprehend marketing material. Sports bodies should avoid over-stylising their injury claims. However, injury data should still be accessible and presented in a manner that the general population can understand.

(d) Cultivating a critical attitude towards claims that are made by spokespeople: This proposal relates to the established cultural habits of injury reporting by sports bodies. Rather than trying to persuade potential participants and parents how safe a sport is, it should become good practice in sports bodies to acknowledge that many other sports might well be less injurious to participants.

While it is important to recognise that risk of injury is inherent to all sports, claims that trivialise risk might also be present in narratives which frames the acceptance of risk as an inherent part of life. For example, Roger Goodell, the NFL Commissioner remarked that there "There's risk in life. There's risk sitting on the couch" (Gutierrez, 2016). Similarly, the Rugby England CEO Ian Ritchie remarked "It's about the proportionality of risk. There's still a risk if you try and cross the road or go on a car trip up the M1 [motorway]; that's another important message we need to get out" (Mairs, 2016). If proportionality of risk is indeed important, consumers must have access to such information. Acknowledging that the risk in collision sports might be higher than other sports is good ethical practice.

Conclusion

This chapter attempted to explore connections between corporate motivations and the framing of injury risk. This is not to say these were discrete stages. There was certainly overlap between the roles as the chronology has unfolded. The process could best be thought of as iterative, with ongoing reflection over time and interplay between the roles of academic as analyst, advocate and theorist.

Regarding the aspect of RT which does not allege a greenwashing conspiracy on the part of national governing bodies, academics should remain vigilant about the possibility for such behaviour. Organisations' pecuniary interests might easily spill over into unscrupulous behaviour. The academic community must also be wary of the close connections to the funders of research. At the time of writing, I note with interest a large proportion of injury research published by salaried employees of sports bodies.

A core focus of this chapter was to explore how sports governing bodies of collision sports might distort injury and risk data in marketing material. This analysis exposes troubling behaviours emanating from some sports governing bodies. By conceiving of sports governing organisations as corporate 'bodies', the analysis diagnoses the distortionary practices as Risk Trivialisation. The analysis suggests that RT can be minimised if sports governing bodies develop a set of critically oriented reflective practices. Many sports have expansionist visions. However, despite much rhetoric about player welfare, safety and evidence-based practice, various sports bodies are both afflicted with RT, and subsequently afflict audiences with inaccurate or false information. It is surely the case that injury data and claims about risk should be carefully constructed, thoroughly checked and judiciously reported. Consumers, potential participants and parents are at least possibly influenced by data to make decisions about what they do, buy and participate in. By describing and analysing Risk Trivialisation, it would be beneficial for all if more due diligence is applied in the reporting of injury statistics in all sports, in order to promote informed participation.

It is notable that a recent article by Quarrie *et al.* (2017) has claimed that "based on the evidence currently available, the risks to children playing rugby do not appear to be inordinately high compared with those in a range of other childhood sports and activities" (p. 1134). Another article in the same issue of the same journal concluded that a "cautionary approach requires the removal of the tackle from school rugby as the quickest and most effective method of reducing high injury rates in youth rugby, a public health priority" (Pollock *et al.*, 2017). While the debate about the acceptable level of risk in collision sport continues, what is surely non-negotiable is the misleading of the public. While appreciating that knowledge about injury is socially constructed, the accepted scientific canon of measurement must not be corrupted. The trivialisation of risk in sports with high injury rates is surely something that the parents, participants and governing bodies should not ignore.

References

ACC (2016). Sporting claim statistics 2010–2014. Retrieved from www.acc.co.nz/about-acc/statistics/

Advertising Standards Authority for Ireland (2016). The Essence of Good Advertising. Retrieved from www.asai.ie/

Arnason, A., Sigurdsson, S.B., Gudmundsson, A., Holme, I., Engebretsen, L. and Bahr, R. (2004). Physical fitness, injuries, and team performance in soccer. *Medicine and Science in Sport and Exercise*, *36*, 278–285.

Beck, U. (1992). From industrial society to the risk society: Questions of survival, social structure and ecological enlightenment. *Theory, Culture & Society*, *9*(1), 97–123.

Brooks, J.H.M., Fuller, C.W., Kemp, S.P.T. and Reddin, R.B. (2005). Epidemiology of injuries in English professional rugby union: part 1 – match injuries. *British Journal of Sports Medicine*, *39*, 757–766.

Dahlström, Ö., Jacobsson, J. and Timpka, T. (2015). Overcoming the organization–practice barrier in sports injury prevention: A nonhierarchical organizational model. *Scandinavian Journal of Medicine and Science in Sports*, *25*, e414–e422.

Dunning, E. (2008). Sport as a male preserve: Notes on the social sources of masculine identity and its transformations. In N. Elias and E. Dunning (eds), *Quest for Excitement: Sport and Leisure in the Civilising Process (The Collected Works of Norbert Elias)*, vol. 7 (pp. 242–259). Dublin: UCD Press.

England Rugby (2012). Seizing the opportunity: The RFU Strategic Plan 2012/13-2016/17. Retrieved from www.englandrugby.com/mm/Document/General/General/01/30/47/26/RFU_Strategic_Plan_2013_2017_Neutral.pdf

England Rugby (2016a). About CBRE All Schools. Retrieved from www.englandrugby.com/about-the-rfu/all-schools/about-all-schools

England Rugby (2016b). Rugby safe. Retrieved from www.englandrugby.com/rugbysafe/

England Rugby (2017). Primary staff development. Retrieved from www.england rugby.com/my-rugby/education/schools/primary/staff-development/

Federal Trade Commission (2016). Truth in advertising. Retrieved from www.ftc.gov/news-events/media-resources/truth-advertising

Finch, C., Owen, N. and Price, R. (2001). Current injury or disability as a barrier to being more physically active. *Medicine and Science in Sport and Exercise*, *33*, 778–782.

Finch, C. (2006). A new framework for research leading to sports injury prevention. *Journal of Science and Medicine in Sport*, *9*, 3–9.

Fortington, L.V., van der Worp, H., van den Akker-Scheek, I. and Finch, C.F. (2017). Reporting multiple individual injuries in studies of team ball sports: A systematic review of current practice. *Sports Medicine*. doi: 10.1007/s40279-016-0637-3

Fuller, C.W. (2008). Catastrophic injury in rugby union: Is the level of risk acceptable? *Sports Medicine*, *38*, 975–986.

Fuller, C. and Drawer, S. (2004). The application of risk management in sport. *Sports Medicine*, *34*(6), 349–356.

Gutierrez, P. (2016). Roger Goodell: If I had son, I'd 'love' to have him play football. Retrieved from www.espn.co.uk/nfl/story/_/id/14722212/roger-goodell-says-had-son-love-play-football

Hume, P.A., Theadom, A., Lewis, G.N., Quarrie, K.L., Brown, S.R, Hill, R. and Marshall, S.W. (2016). A comparison of cognitive function in former rugby union players compared with former non-contact-sport players and the impact of concussion history. *Sports Medicine*, *47*(6), 1209–1220.

Kreisfeld, R., Harrison, J.E., Pointer, S. and AIHW (2014, 4 November). Australian Sports Injury Hospitalisations 2011–12. Injury research and statistics series no. 92. Cat. no. INJCAT 168. Canberra: Australian Institute of Health and Welfare. Retrieved from www.aihw.gov.au/publication-detail/?id=60129549100

Liston, K., McDowell, M., Malcolm, M., Scott-Bell, A. and Waddington, I. (2016) On being 'head strong': The pain zone and concussion in non-elite rugby union. *International Review for the Sociology of Sport*. doi: 10.1177/101269 0216679966

Mairs, G. (2016). Fear of rise in concussion cases after former Saracens captain Alistair Hargreaves forced to retire. *Telegraph*. Retrieved from www.telegraph.co.uk/rugby-union/2016/10/05/saracens-captain-alistair-hargreaves-forced-into-retirement-afte/

Nicholl, J.P., Coleman, P. and Williams, B.T. (1995). The epidemiology of sports and exercise related injury in the United Kingdom. *British Journal of Sports Medicine*, *29*(4), 232–238.

Nyiri P. (2015). Re: The unknown risks of youth rugby. *British Medical Journal*. Retrieved from www.bmj.com/content/350/bmj.h26/rr-9

Omalu, B. (2016). Don't let kids play football. *New York Times*. Retrieved from www.nytimes.com/2015/12/07/opinion/dont-let-kids-play-football.html?_r=0

Physical Activity Expert Group [PAEG] (2016). Response to Sports Collision Injury Collective (SCIC) Letter for UK CMOs. Retrieved from www.sportcic. com/

Piggin, J. and Pollock, A. (2016). World Rugby's erroneous and misleading representation of Australian sports' injury statistics. *British Journal of Sports Medicine*, *51*, 1108.

Piggin, J. and Bairner, A. (2017). An urgent call for clarity regarding England Rugby's injury claims. *Idrotts Forum.* Retrieved from http://idrottsforum.org/feature-piggin-bairner170523/

Piggin, J. and Bairner, A. (2018). What counts as 'the evidence'? A need for an urgent review of injury risk in school rugby. *British Journal of Sports Medicine*, *53*, 10–11.

Pollock, A.M., White, A.J. and Kirkwood, G. (2017). Evidence in support of the call to ban the tackle and harmful contact in school rugby: A response to World Rugby. *British Journal of Sports Medicine*, *51*, 1113–1117.

Pringle, R.G., McNair, P. and Stanley, S. (1998). Incidence of sporting injury in New Zealand youths aged 6–15 years. *British Journal of Sports Medicine*, *32*, 49–52.

Quarrie, K.L., Brooks, J.H.M., Burger, N., Hume, P.A. and Jackson, S. (2017). Facts and values: On the acceptability of risks in children's sport using the example of rugby: A narrative review. *British Journal of Sports Medicine*, *51*, 1134–1139.

Raftery, M. (2016). Response to: World Rugby's erroneous and misleading representation of Australian sports' injury statistics. *British Journal of Sports Medicine*, 51, 1174.

Roberts, S.P., Trewartha, G., England, M., Goodison, W. and Stokes, K.A. (2017). Concussions and head injuries in English community rugby union match play. *American Journal of Sports Medicine*, Feb:*45*(2), 480–487.

Schwarz, A. (2016). N.F.L.-backed Youth Program says it reduced concussions. The data disagrees. *New York Times*. Retrieved from www.nytimes.com/2016/07/28/sports/football/nfl-concussions-youth-program-heads-up-football.html

SCIC (2016). Open letter: Preventing injuries in children playing school rugby. Retrieved from www.sportcic.com/resources/Open%20Letter%20SportCIC%2

Shrier, I., Steele, R.J., Hanley, J. and Rich, B. (2009). Analyses of injury count data: Some do's and don'ts. *American Journal of Epidemiology*, *170*, 1307–1315.

Sport England (2016). Active People Survey 10 October 2015–September 2016. Retrieved from www.sportengland.org/media/11325/1x30_sport_16plus-factsheet_aps10.pdf

Tucker, R., Raftery, M. and Verhagen, E. (2016). Injury risk and a tackle ban in youth Rugby Union: reviewing the evidence and searching for targeted, effective interventions: A critical review. *British Journal of Sports Medicine*, *50*, 921–925.

UK Chief Medical Officers [UK CMOs] (2016). RE: Open letter: Preventing injuries in children playing school rugby, 2016. Retrieved from www.sportcic.com/resources

USA Football (2014). USA Football 2014 Annual Report. Retrieved from https://usafootball.com/sites/default/files/uploads/usafbannual_2014.pdf

USA Football (2016). Heads Up Football. Retrieved from https://usafootball.com/programs/heads-up-football/

van Mechelen, W., Hlobil, H. and Kemper, H.C. (1992). Incidence, severity, aetiology and prevention of sports injuries: A review of concepts. *British Journal of Sports Medicine*, *14*(2), 82–99.

World Rugby (2014). Strategic Plan background. Retrieved from www.worldrugby.org/strategic-plan?lang=en

World Rugby (2016a). Response to 'Ban on Rugby Tackling' Petition in the UK. 2 March.

World Rugby (2016b). Player welfare: Putting players first. Retrieved from http://playerwelfare.worldrugby.org/

World Rugby (2016c). Strategic Plan. Retrieved from http://pulse-static-files.s3.amazonaws.com/worldrugby/document/2016/09/06/26664bae-4b24-4622-901c-c094666a2a96/2016-2020_Strategic_Plan_English.pdf

9 Conclusion
People, power and possibilities

At the beginning of this book I framed physical activity as inherently political and proposed a definition of physical activity as

> the idea of human movement as a **means** by which an array of political, educational, nationalistic, health, environmental, commercial and personal goals are operationalised, enacted, reinforced and hoped for by institutional and individual bodies.

Through the chapters within this volume, I have attempted to:

- examine how physical activity policy and promotion is inherently political,
- show how physical activity has been consciously and politically connected with a wide variety of other social arenas,
- interrogate some of the dominant ideas which inform thinking about physical activity,
- examine the use and usefulness of different forms of evidence in physical activity policy,
- examine the paradoxes and tensions about physical activity policy and promotion which arise in this multifaceted domain, and
- illuminate the potentially problematic effects that interventions can have on individuals and the possible implications for future settings.

The various case studies presented here offer insight into the politics of physical activity, yet it is clear there is a multitude of swirling issues and conflicts about people's opportunities to be active, their understandings of what physical activity can and should include, and contests over resource allocation. This is a great multitude of ongoing conflicts, which of course cannot be detailed in one text; everything from the politics of public cycle lockers to cycle superhighways, the politics of which subjects get taught in physical education classes, the politics of which activities are socially acceptable and which are not. One thing I hope that is clear from this book is that physical activity is not neutral. To evoke physical activity and justifications for it is a deeply political act.

So where to from here? Because physical activity is a deeply personal endeavour at an individual level, ideas created by policy come with a particular ethical responsibility beyond making people 'more' active. For example, the WHO mentions "culturally appropriate" activity. What might that mean for people and groups who want to transcend or transgress dominant notions of activity in their own communities? Should public protest, as one form of physical transgression, be promoted or suppressed? Is it possible for marginalised groups to resist oppression without being culturally inappropriate?

Some general thoughts are offered below for different readers of this book.

For **undergraduate students** reading this text I encourage you to question the assumptions of the models you are presented with, as I did with Nike's model in Chapter 7. Ask who wrote the text and what interests they have. (Yes, including me!). Ask your lecturers if you can do 'real world' assignments on the communities you grew up in and which you know about.

For **postgraduate students** conducting research into physical activity promotion, consider vested interests, and make your default setting suspicion about 'industry funding'. There have been too many cases of commercial enterprises targeting children, using the Trojan horse of health promotion to flaunt their junk food wares to children. Research how to break structural inequalities and how to lobby and advocate effectively. There might not be funding to do this, but it is very important.

For **academic colleagues** who read this book, thank you for your time! Encourage your students to critique the model I offer here. Let them dismantle it and create something better in its place.

Policy makers, I do not envy you. Limited budgets, limited insight and limited time all conspire to end in policy of limited effect, and programme evaluations which often show small, temporary gains, if anything at all. If the problem of physical activity is so severe, this is surely the time for radical action. I hope the cases provided here encourage reflection about how things can be done differently.

For **all of us**, on the matter of policy creation and programme implementation, we should be very careful about conflating the reasons for physical activity with the benefits of physical activity. These are often distinctly different things.

We should all ask ourselves the best way to critique organisations which are already critiquing the status quo and dominant power structures (such as corporations, academic societies and states). Shouldn't we all be fighting the same battles against sedentary living and unhealthy lifestyles? Well, there is a clear need to consider the interests at work. Both commercial and ideological incentives need to be critiqued and exposed, whether that is the over-competitiveness in youth sport, or the targeting of youth to promote junk food through sport, or state surveillance of citizens and residents which impinges of their dignity and liberty.

What is a utopian vision of physical activity around the world? Is it everybody active, every day? I would say no, since the freedom to be inactive is more important than any incentive to be active. My own values of physical activity promotion are to facilitate personal human expression through physical activity (which does not cause harm to others). Whether or not these activities meet thresholds of risk reduction is not sufficient rationale for me. The aim should be individual expression through human movement, not meeting medicalised notions of fitness and health. This is in line with the notion of minimising domination discussed in Chapter 2.

The future of physical activity politics

Chapter 3 offered a theoretical framework on how physical activity is being operationalised as a powerful policy issue. The theory was preluded by the idea that it is not sufficient to accept the rationalities that physical activity interest groups and promoters offer as the totality of understanding of physical activity, since this buys in to the meanings and values of that specific interest group. By examining assumptions in policy proclamations, omissions, subtleties, we can contribute to minimising various forms of domination. Zanker and Gard explain why it is necessary to do this:

> The idea that physical activity means different things to different people hardly needs to be reiterated. And yet it is surely part of the ongoing role of scholarship to map and probe the evolving meanings of physical activity and people's experiences of it. It is important for scholarship to do this for many reasons, but perhaps most important of all is the need to offer narratives that run counter to dominant ways of thinking about physical activity … counter-narratives are important because they highlight the ways in which powerful cultural, political, and economic forces sometimes serve to narrow our understandings and experiences of physical activity.
>
> (Zanker and Gard, 2008, p. 48)

So greater scrutiny of differences between the promoted *benefits* of physical activity must be discussed in tandem with the *reasons* people are physically active. These are not necessarily always the same thing. To reiterate, I am sure most health promoters are benevolent people who are slowly but surely trying to make positive change happen. However, we should all remind ourselves that physical activity is a deeply personal endeavour for each person, and spaces for promoting physical activity should not be places of potential exploitation, whether it is commercial exploitation or dominant ideological impositions.

There are two aspects of resistance worth mentioning. The first is resistance of people and groups that constrain or prohibit the fulfilment of physically active lives. The second is resistance and questioning of the policies that attempt to create a specific sort of active population – one which is overly surveilled, one in which activity is promoted to meet commercial or nationalistic ends rather than humanistic goals, or one in which shame is used to encourage people to be active. Resistance is needed by all people. Zanker and Gard wrote that "There is simply no significant opposing force to the moral and scientific logic of modern physical activity" (2008, p. 59). We can all be that opposing force.

Some of the chapters in the book may be perceived as being overly critical. However, criticality and resistance can be 'healthy' parts of the health promotion process. Keeping in line with the sentiments throughout this book, I believe that resistance is an engagement with the policy process, and can be conceived of as productive; it is "an integral part of and contributor to programs regarded as successful, and [may] be incorporated into programs rather than merely acting as an external source of program failure" (O'Malley, 1996, p. 313).

Above all, this book has endeavoured to show that physical activity is not simply "any bodily movement produced by skeletal muscles that requires energy expenditure" (WHO, 2018). It is much more than that.

References

O'Malley, P. (1996). Indigenous governance. *Economy and Society*, 25(3), 310–326.

WHO (2018). Global Action Plan on Physical Activity 2018–2030: More active people for a healthier world. World Health Organisation, Geneva.

Zanker, C. and Gard, M. (2008). Fatness, fitness, and the moral universe of sport and physical activity. *Sociology of Sport Journal*, 25(1), 48–65.

Index

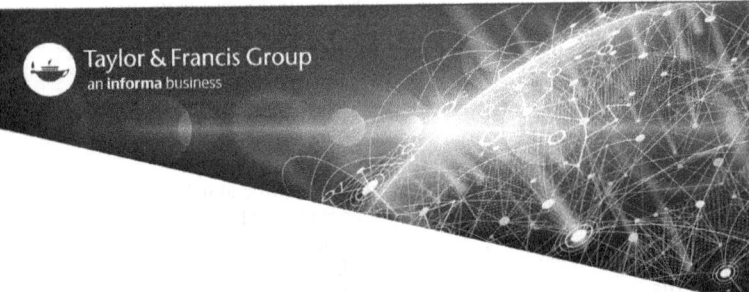
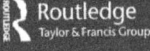
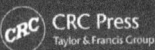